Spiritual Portraits of the Energy Release Points

A Compendium of Acupuncture Point Messages Found Within the 12 Meridians and the 8 Extraordinary Vessels

Michele Marie Gervais B.A B.Ed

Tellwell Talent
www.tellwell.ca

ISBNs:
Hardcover: 978-1-77302-005-1
Paperback: 978-1-77302-003-7
eBook: 978-1-77302-004-4

This book is dedicated to
My Three Treasures

Foreword

My name is Natalie Jensen. I'm a Doctor of Traditional Chinese Medicine, Registered Acupuncturist and Registered Massage Therapist. I'm honoured and appreciative to be a student and a good friend of Michele Marie Gervais. I was introduced to Michele by a friend who was interested in healing her animals through sound. Michele has developed a healing system called Soundtouch Therapy - Esoteric Vibrational Sound Healing, which explores the effects of sound and colour vibration in healing the body. Michele has an incredibly angelical presence and the gifts she brings to you are like no other. She performs a level of healing which moves your heart into a state of bliss along your soul's journey. The gifts she shares with you, through this book will touch the depths of your soul.

Soundtouch Therapy (Esoteric Vibrational Sound Healing), connects one with the universe. Each fork is turned to the vibration and sound frequency of the planets as well as to the frequency of healthy organs. Sound produces colour, and further work is done to enhance the functioning and flow of energy. Healing is done through the Acupuncture meridian system, the Chakra system and the etheric body. Like each Acupuncture point, each sound frequency has a certain function and indication. Based on a Chinese Medicine diagnosis, the points and forks are picked according to the ailment the person is dealing with. It can be emotional, mental and/or physical. The combination of all the therapies, including the Spiritual portrait of the Energy Release Point (Acupuncture point), make a beautiful plethora of a conscious connection, through the body, mind and spirit.

The Compendium of Energy Release Points that Michele has created, is an incredible tool that one can use in their everyday life. It is a book meant to be on every bookshelf, healer or self-healer. I have personally had the opportunity to connect with these Energy Release Points for my own healing. The level of creativity, connection and depth these Energy Release Points express, far exceeds any other materials I have used. I resonate so much with these points because they directly relate to the Acupuncture meridian system. All the points are coordinated with the organs and systems in our body. The Energy Release Points are precise and to the point, with an in depth explanation that accesses many levels, or should I say an esoteric compilation of enhanced Acupuncture points. An example that comes to mind is when you have a distinctive memory that triggers your olfactory senses. You remember where you were, what you were doing, and how you felt in that moment all by remembering that smell. The Energy Release Points are that powerful. Whatever is going on in your life whether you are fully conscious of it or not, the Energy Release Points will trigger what you need to know. It helps in finding direction, brings ease and grace, it allows your mind, body and soul to cleanse and purify you. The Energy Release Points will help guide you and find purpose in your everyday life and in every step of your way. Stop, think, take a moment, a deep breath in. Look at what is truly troubling your soul. It may be time to open up and continue to learn what is underlying in you. This book provides a key or tool to help in the understanding of your journey.

I have incorporated the Energy Release Points and other techniques of Soundtouch Therapy into my Acupuncture and Massage practice. I use it for clients who need more than just a physical release and for those who want to know why the pain in their body isn't going away easily. By opening up the points and awakening to the understanding of the pain, it allows for healing on a deeper level. It brings awareness, epiphanies, and a greater understanding of what one needs to know, that one wasn't sure of before.

Michele Marie Gervais was guided to open up your Soul's journey through these powerful Energy Release Points. They are here to elevate, alleviate and connect you to the work being used with Colourtouch, Soundtouch, Flower Essence Therapy, acupressure, acupuncture and reflexology. May this work assist you in your work, and may your work guide you to where you need to be. May the presence of the Divine connect to your Soul's true Essence.

Dr. Natalie Jensen TCMD, R.Ac, R.M.T.

Preface

This work is presented for information purposes and is not meant to be used as a guide for diagnosing and/or treating medical and psychological/mental issues. In those instances where medical assistance may be required, it is recommended to seek advice and treatment from a qualified, licensed physician.

The intention and purpose of this book is to enhance and broaden the scope of healing: acupuncture, acupressure, Soundtouch* Therapy, Colourtouch, Flower Essence Therapy as well as practitioners of new modalities in energy healing, and all those interested in self healing. This is also a book which integrates Ancient Wisdom with new information of this age. It is healing through spirituality, for spirituality is the means through which one learns to know oneself. To understand and discover who you are and why you are here. This book can also be used as a tool in the elevation and expansion of consciousness through Inner Plane work as well as opening and anchoring positive light frequencies into our full body systems. It is not meant to be religious in view, however, it is intended to introduce and present philosophical ideals and to raise consciousness.

I invite you to read in the spirit of openness, remembering that truths present as a many-sided jewel, different aspects perceived at different times. The use of these Energy Release Points is to create a healing environment precisely through conscious connection to the Essence of the Spirit of the Energy Release Points. It is then this conscious connection that energetically impacts the energy fields, energy bodies and the subtle bodies which, in turn, influence whole body systems and physical well-being. This action is understood through the science of quantum physics and the energy and phenomena of resonance and vibration. This is truly vibrational healing at a very profound level.

The illustrations used in this book are artistic representations and are not meant to be an anatomical reference. For those who wish to know the exact location of an Energy Release Point, there are excellent point location books/cards available, such as Deadman, Peter & Mazin Al Khafaji w/ Kevin Baker. A Manual of Acupuncture.

A note about the names of the Energy Release Channels. There has always been question as to how to translate Chinese symbols into the English language and still grasp the meaning of the pictogram. I have chosen to translate San Jiao as the Three Elixir Fields as they refer to energetic cavities where transformational alchemical fire can be accessed. The Ren is a yin vessel of conception and creation, therefore the name Divine Feminine Matrix is appropriate. The Du is a yang expression of governance, hence the name Divine Masculine Director. In keeping with the feminine and masculine etymology of yin and yang and the purpose of the motility vessels (assisting movement) and linking vessels (assisting the strengthening of connecting structures) the names Yin/Yang Qiao Mai is translated as Feminine/Masculine Vessel of Movement and Yin/Yang Wei Mai is translated as Feminine/Masculine Vessel of Structure.

I acknowledge Hans Cousto for his pioneering work in measuring cosmic frequencies and the harmonic relationship which exists between the cosmos and the general structure of all beings. His insights of using sound to heal via the application of tuning forks on the acupuncture points of the body is truly inspirational. It is with sincere expressions of gratitude that I wish to thank my dear friend Dixie Dash for her tireless editing, commitment and encouragement throughout the process of bringing this book into being. Dr. Natalie Jensen for sharing and integrating the Energy Release Points within her acupuncture clinic. Sabina Schmid for bringing her talents and amazing insights into the creation of the beautiful illustrations and cover art. My many teachers along my journey, notably Inge Knott and Michel Green. My clients and students who enthusiastically spurred me onwards out of necessity for their personal healing. I am grateful for my husband Lambert Bordeaux for his tireless proofreading as well as for his active support in holding space for me to manifest this project. Lastly, I wish to acknowledge my daughters: Christina, Sophia and Larisa for their encouragement and enthusiastic support.

* Soundtouch Therapy is a holistic modality created by the author. It integrates the vibrational frequencies of sound, light and colour to support the healing of the physical, emotional, mental and spiritual bodies. In a therapeutic session, a precise treatment protocol is designed to address the concerns of the individual. Sound, colour and light are applied to the body via the energy field, energy body, energy centres (chakras), Energy Release Channels (meridians) and Energy Release Points (acupuncture points). Soundtouch is a therapy that is effective on it's own or as a complementary therapy. The resulting experience is unique to each individual. To learn more about private sessions, sound for self healing workshops or the practitioner certification program, please visit www.harmonic-medicine.com.

How To Use This Book

This book is intended to be used as a tool for understanding and bringing awareness to the environment that created the condition for an imbalance to manifest as a disharmony, (dis-ease) within one's physical, emotional, mental or spiritual well-being. For acupuncturists and those trained in Chinese Medicine, this book can be used to enhance the healing of your patients. Patients may read through the virtues and disharmonies to bring conscious awareness to their situation before their acupuncture treatment. For those new to acupuncture, this book lends very well to pendulum dowsing, body dowsing or random opening and picking as there will be a message for the inquirer.

The quest for identification of an appropriate Energy Release Point is to usually answer a question in regards to an issue that one is facing. (This question can be in regards to work done in Colourtouch or Soundtouch Therapy. This question can also be a curiosity as to why an acupuncturist would choose a certain acupuncture point over another.) It is important to identify a key soul issue. For example: there can be a manifestation of physical issues surrounding the digestive system. It would be appropriate to first choose the Energy Release Channel of the Stomach and then choose an Energy Release Point pertaining to that channel. This can be a starting point. The questioning process in itself is a way to root out an imbalance in the self healing process and contributes greatly to establishing the proper conditions for the answer to present itself.

It is important to consider that the messages of the Energy Release Points reflect the experiences of each individual: past and present. This is to say that many times we have an experience from the past that still affects the flow of energy in an Energy Release Point, or Energy Release Channel, in the present. It is important to note that an Energy Release Point that is not flowing optimally or considered blocked, will impact the health and well-being of an individual should it not be addressed. When working with an acupuncturist, or through acupressure or reflexology, the stimulation of the point either through manipulation or a needle, will unblock the point. The conscious connection with the Energy Release Point will amplify the positive effects of the healing. For those who are working towards self healing and are in between visits with their health therapist or who are simply self guiding their healing process, intention, visualization and prayer are very powerful. A simple invocation to unblock an Energy Release Point is as follows:

"I ask for the Energy Release Point of (insert the name of the Energy Release Point here) to connect with my Energy Body, Energy Field and Physical Consciousness, with the help of the Divine. I ask for the Energy Release Point to assist me with (insert the virtue or a sentence which resonates with you, OR insert the disharmony that you wish to release) I ask for the Energy Release Point of (insert name of the Energy Release Point) to unblock, activate and (place your hands on your temples) to stabilize."

By unblocking and activating an Energy Release Point, one is actually healing an imbalance from the past and this in turn will affect the present and future. This unblocking and activation can also serve to bring up layers of energy that also needs addressing. By bringing up these layers in a conscious manner, they are more actively transformed and released.

Finally, the portraits of the Energy Release Points reflect the Universal Law of Polarity. The dualistic aspects will be presented as Virtues and as

Disharmonies. This is done so that upon recognition of the two opposites, one finds harmony and equanimity through balance.

It is my hope that this compendium of Energy Release Points serve the reader well in their quest for self healing, as well as enrich the modality of healing for those in a clinical practice. Let this publication serve as a resource for deeper awareness and understanding for the challenges one faces in their journey through life.

Michele Marie Gervais B.A B.Ed
mgcreate@gmail.com
Creator of Soundtouch Therapy
Esoteric Vibrational Sound Healing

Table of Contents

What are Energy Release Channels

Energy Release Channels are streams of energy that are situated on top of the Energy Body and flow through a casing of light. There are twelve familiar Energy Release Channels and eight Extraordinary Energy Release Channels.

List of the Twelve Familiar Energy Release Channels

LUNG
URINARY BLADDER
LARGE INTESTINE
KIDNEY
STOMACH
PERICARDIUM
SPLEEN
THREE ELIXIR FIELDS *(Triple Burner or Triple Heater)*
HEART
GALLBLADDER
SMALL INTESTINE
LIVER

Function of the Energy Release Channels

These Energy Release Channels allow for the movement and flow of energy through a network of beams of light in the full body systems. There are energies from one's thoughts, feelings and actions that are stored in the energy fields of organs, glands, muscles and bones. When these energies are brought to awareness and are healed, the body systems are no longer required to hold on to them. The Energy Release Channels then release the old and bring in higher vibrational energies to circulate throughout the body activating the body's self healing abilities. If energy that is leaving the energy system has an interruption of flow and is subsequently blocked, pain will be manifested. If energy is constantly being released and the inflow of higher vibrational energy is either blocked from entering; unable to be circulated within the body systems; or if the body systems cannot hold the light frequency; again, pain may be manifested as well as emotional/mental/spiritual disharmonies are likely to occur.

List of the Eight Extraordinary Energy Release Channels

(The Chinese name and translation of these energy release channels are in brackets)

DIVINE FEMININE MATRIX *(Ren - Conception Vessel)*
DIVINE MASCULINE DIRECTOR *(Du- Governor Vessel)*
THE PENETRATING INTERFACE *(Chong - Penetrating Vessel)*
THE VESSEL OF GUIDANCE *(Dai Mai - Girdle Vessel)*
FEMININE VESSEL OF MOVEMENT *(Yin Qiao Motility/Stepping vessel)*
MASCULINE VESSEL OF MOVEMENT *(Yang Qiao Motility/Stepping vessel)*
FEMININE VESSEL OF STRUCTURE *(Yin Wei Linking/Heel vessel)*
MASCULINE VESSEL OF STRUCTURE *(Yang Wei Linking/Heel vessel)*

These vessels are the streams of energy that are responsible for the creation of the Twelve Energy Release Channels and as such they connect to the original cells of creation of all the bodies, body systems and sensory systems. They are represented by the movement of spirit and represent an aspect of the Creative Force. They are sometimes seen as cosmic energies emerging from a vortex of energy that come to a point at the centre of our being. They are the powers of life - the generative force of the Universal ALL. It is from this centre that the cosmic energies change, transmute, merge and radiate in the concentric systems which form the basis of the body of Light. The blueprint for the physical. They govern the lifestream as it plays out on the physical, emotional, mental and spiritual planes. They represent the movement and structure of the Divine Feminine and the Divine Masculine. They connect to the original source of all life.

In Soundtouch Therapy we use the energy of Sound to move through and harmonize these eight original vessels of creation to strengthen their ability to harmonize the Energy Release Channels in order to create wholeness, harmony and balance in the full body systems including the sensory systems. This enables the entire physical body to tap into its own self healing abilities, as well as regenerate and rejuvenate because of its communication with the other metaphysical bodies. In combination with the healing therapy of Colourtouch, one can rebuild the body as well as slow and reverse the aging process.

It is important to correct all the breakdowns in the Energy Release Channels. This is done through the unblocking and activation of Energy Release Points.

What are Energy Release Points?

Energy Release Points are little vortexes of energy that are part of the Energy Release Channels. The movement of the Energy Release Points are subtle, however, they address profound imbalances which occur on the physical, emotional/mental and spiritual levels. The purpose of Energy Release Points are to release energy as well as bring new energy in. Each Energy Release Point has a specific, deeper meaning which is connected to the physical, emotional, mental and spiritual aspects of the body. These Energy Release Points are constantly flowing energy through the movement of the vortex, however, sometimes because of life experiences, these Points may become blocked or constricted in their ability to flow energy, causing an imbalance or disharmony to show up in one or more of our body systems. These imbalances can be re-harmonized by using mind/heart consciousness to connect with the spirit of the energy in the point. This re-harmonization is followed by exploring and understanding the reason behind the imbalance and then asking it to unblock and activate. Understanding the issue and the message of the spirit of the Energy Release Point is key to personal self healing and empowerment. These Energy Release Points can also be further treated physically should one choose to explore acupuncture or acupressure healing techniques. Ultimately, the goal is to evolve in our understanding of how we create the imbalances within our energy, in order to re-harmonize the body to health and wellness.

SECTION 1

Brief Summary of Each of the
Energy Release Channels

Energy Release Channel of the Lung

The inherent energy of the Lungs is to receive spirit, the inspirations which regulate the quality of life. It holds the energy of the Divine Masculine which is strongly supported by the Divine Feminine. The Divine Masculine provides the catalyst to spark the fire of transformation while the support of the Divine Feminine holds the energy as seeds filled with potential to nourish the passions of the heart. The Lungs surround the heart and therefore minister to the energy of guidance from the promptings of Spirit as inspired from the Creative Force. This ensures that life is prolific, abundant and inspired, assuring the presence of vitality needed for Soul growth and evolution.

When the Lung is out of harmony there is rigidity, inflexibility and hopelessness.

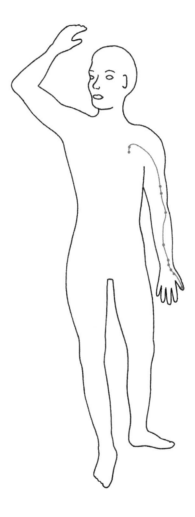

List of Energy Release Points for the Energy Release Channel of the Lung

Energy Release Channel of the Large Intestine

The inherent energy of the Large Intestine is that of transportation and transformation of the inessential in order to be able to receive the new. It functions in partnership with the lungs and represents the breath of the Universal energy as represented by the 5th universal law which states "The ALL is Rhythm". The mucosa and submucosa hold on to emotions and it is necessary to allow emotions to flow. The Large Intestine is also responsible for releasing the energy of old belief systems which is a necessity in the creation of a new life.

When the Large Intestine is out of harmony everything is blocked or carelessly released without discernment.

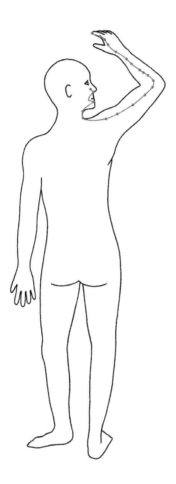

List of Energy Release Points for the Energy Release Channel of the Large Intestine

Energy Release Channel of the Stomach

The inherent energy of the Stomach provides the space to balance and alchemically harmonize the physical, emotional, mental and spiritual bodies as embodied within the central, main and core channels of the energy body. It represents the vitality of nourishment of our perceptions of experience as presented in all aspects of life. (In past, present, parallel and potential future life). It holds the energy of the Divine Feminine and is supported by the Divine Masculine energy allowing us to of follow our path with stability.

When the Stomach is out of harmony there is disconnection with the Earth, leading to insecurity, instability, confusion and distress.

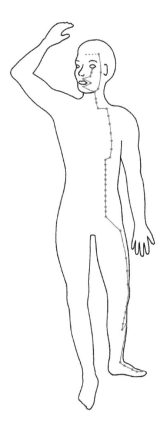

List of Energy Release Points for the Energy Release Channel of the Stomach

Energy Release Channel of the Spleen

The inherent energy of the Spleen is that of storage and distribution of vitality through a complex transportation system bringing nourishment throughout the body via the circulatory and lymphatic systems. This nourishment has strong vital energy which can penetrate every cell, giving the body it's ability to move. It's purposeful question is "How may I serve?". It works in direct partnership with the Stomach, adding the qualities of humility, balance, security and stability.

When the Spleen is out of harmony there is exhaustion, fatigue, struggle and depletion in the full body systems.

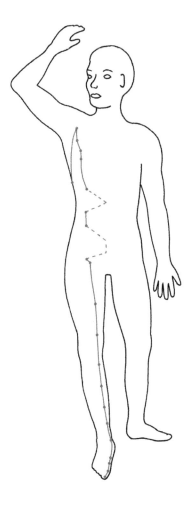

List of Energy Release Points for the Energy Release Channel of the Spleen

Energy Release Channel of the Heart

The inherent energy of the Heart is that of our I AM Presence and therefore our inner divinity. It is foundational to Being and needs to remain open in order to receive loving wisdom from our Essence as connected to the Creative Force. It embodies wisdom, peace and calmness. It is the embodiment of love, and through love can circulate divine energy throughout all the Energy Release Channels so that the body works harmoniously to exude the energy of peace, joy, compassion, radiance and revitalization.

When the heart is out of harmony, it shows as excessive laughter and false emotionality.

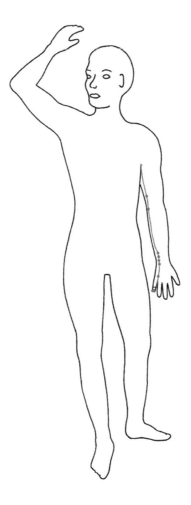

List of Energy Release Points for the Energy Release Channel of the Heart

Energy Release Channel of the Small Intestine

The inherent energy of the Small Intestine is the energy of discernment and sorting. It clearly can ascertain what is beneficial and what is not. It can sort in order to keep what is optimum and release all that is extraneous. It can be likened to a well organized office manager and sometimes it is referred to as the brain of the physical body. However it is the use of alchemy that helps in the transformation and sorting process. Nourishing energy is sent to the heart for circulation to the body, extraneous and non-beneficial elements (both physical and non physical) are sent to the large intestine for elimination.

A Small Intestine that is out of harmony cannot connect with clarity and loses the ability to discern or discriminate.

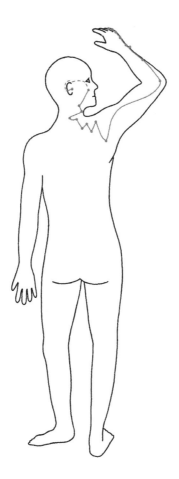

List of Energy Release Points for the Energy Release Channel of the Small Intestine

Energy Release Channel of the Urinary Bladder

The Urinary Bladder is the longest Energy Release Channel. It holds a magnificent reservoir of vitality that is capable of nourishing the body with the life force of water. Our physical body is made mostly of water, it is one of the elemental building blocks of life. This is why SOUND is one of the most effective vehicles to heal the body. Sound travels four times more quickly in water than in the air. The energy of the Urinary Bladder is that of endurance, motivation, ambition, determination to see things through as well as carrying the codes of genetic energy which we can choose to transform. The power of the water element allows for circulation and fluidity of movement.

When the Urinary Bladder is out of harmony we feel lifeless, dry and uncreative. Or we can feel out of control and dispersed.

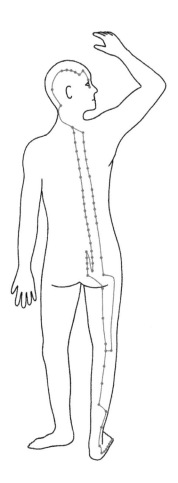

List of Energy Release Points for the Energy Release Channel of the Urinary Bladder

Energy Release Channel of the Kidney

The Kidney works in partnership with the Urinary Bladder. The energy of the Kidneys is similar to the role of a wise and honoured teacher. The Kidneys empower the movement of water and hold the keys to genetic memories. From here stem will, purpose, vitality, strength and creativity. The ability to connect to the wisdom of the jewels of past experiences, heal relationship and imbalances learned through the genetic lineage form the energetics of the Kidney.

When the Kidney is out of harmony there is fear, feelings of being unrooted, lack of vitality, strength and creativity.

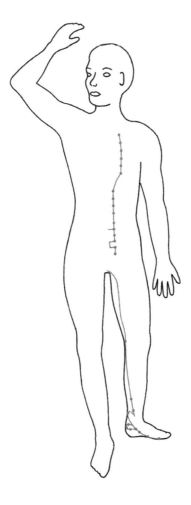

List of Energy Release Points for the Energy Release Channel of the Kidney

Energy Release Channel
of the Pericardium

The inherent energy of the Pericardium is that of creating a sacred circle around the heart. The circle serves to protect the divinity within one's Being. Representatives of this circle: the virtues of trust, wisdom, generosity, compassion, understanding and love, are responsible for carrying out desires and passions. These appropriate actions manifest the vibrations of joy, calm and radiance of Light within the cellular structure of one's Being.

A pericardium out of harmony cannot trust, is narcissistic, dispassionate and misunderstands the intentions of others.

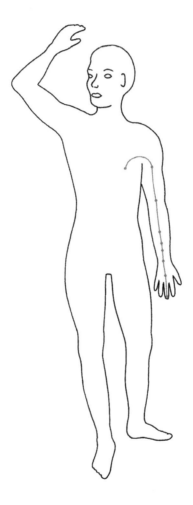

List of Energy Release Points for the Energy Release Channel of the Pericardium

Energy Release Channel of the Three Elixir Fields

The inherent energy of the Three Elixir Fields is that of being the mediator and harmonizing the body in wholeness for it to function at optimum efficiency. This Energy Release Channel connects to the Environmental Part of our energy fields and regulates the inner and outer conditions of life. This regulation is essential in order to live in harmony and balance with what is and with what comes.

When the Three Elixir Fields are out of harmony, we become polarized. Physically this can present as being too hot and too cold at the same time in different parts of the body. On the emotional/mental/spiritual levels this can manifest as conflict.

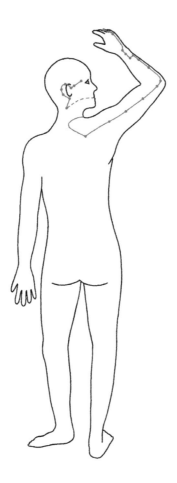

List of Energy Release Points for the Energy Release Channel of the Three Elixir Fields

Energy Release Channel
of the Gallbladder

The inherent energy of the Gallbladder is that of the embodiment of courage in the flesh. It means bravery, courage and the ability to make decisions, give direction of these decisions into precise goals and to purposefully follow through with positive action. The energy also embodies discernment, integrity and justice. Positive action with strength, flexibility, grounded enthusiasm and optimism. It is an overcomer of obstacles.

When the Gallbladder is out of harmony we have conflict, indecision and the feelings of irritation.

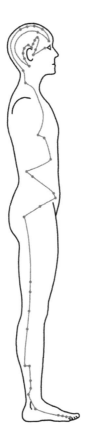

List of Energy Release Points for the Energy Release Channel of the Gallbladder

Energy Release Channel of the Liver

The inherent energy of the Liver is the energy of the Soul's vision and purpose. It is the energy of the Master Planner - the Supreme All Knowing. It is through the liver that we can connect to the master blueprint of life direction, refining our Essence to become who we are meant to be regardless of whatever circumstances are brought to us.

When the Liver is out of harmony, we over plan or do not plan. We can feel hopeless and often experience anger. The anger, however, can be positive showing us that something needs to change.

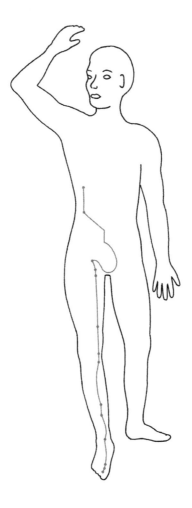

List of Energy Release Points for the Energy Release Channel of the Liver

SECTION 2

Brief Summary of the Extraordinary
Energy Release Channels

(The Chinese name and translation of these Energy Release Channels are in brackets)

Divine Feminine Matrix *(Ren - Conception Vessel)*
Divine Masculine Director *(Du - Governor Vessel)*
The Penetrating Interface *(Chong - Penetrating Vessel)*
The Vessel of Guidance *(Dai Mai - Girdle or Belt Vessel)*
Feminine Vessel of Movement *(Yin Qiao - Yin Motility/Stepping Vessel)*
Masculine Vessel of Movement *(Yang Qiao - Yang Motility/Stepping Vessel)*
Feminine Vessel of Structure *(Yin Wei - Yin Linking/Heel Vessel)*
Masculine Vessel of Structure *(Yang Wei - Yang Linking/Heel Vessel)*

All of the Extraordinary Energy Release Channels have an opening and balancing Energy Release Point. It is through these Energy Release Points that the Extraordinary Energy Release Channel is activated. There are also Energy Release Points within the Extraordinary Energy Release Channel that may be blocked as well and may need attention.

Extraordinary Energy Release Channel of the Divine Feminine Matrix

The Energy Release Channel of the Divine Feminine Matrix is the aspect of the Divine Feminine Energy within the Creative Force which is responsible for co-creation of the physical. It is partnered with the Divine Masculine Energy and work together for creation. It travels in a clockwise energetic pattern of direction. It is, however, responsible for the germination and potential of all existence. It is the vessel through which all life comes. (Although it is the energy of the Divine Masculine that activates and pushes life forward) It is within this matrix that the Creative Force encodes purpose, and it is this connection to purpose that gives Life meaning. The Divine Feminine Matrix is the energy that creates and governs our vital resources, as connected to Soul, through the creation of our etheric and whole body systems. Connection with this Energy Release Channel allows for access to the inner nourishment that is necessary to develop our service along the life path. This Energy Release Channel provides harmony and balance and it alchemically transforms inspiration into creation. It is about the fertility of life.

Disharmonies: *Feelings of being ungrounded, shaky, or fragile; inability to create new ideas; inability to make plans and set goals; fear causing stagnation; apprehension or avoidance of threshold experiences; low self esteem; fear of sexual intimacy; lack of self love. Physical manifestation of night sweating; hot flashes; mental irritability; anxiety; dry mouth at night; dizziness; tinnitus; insomnia; chronic asthma.*

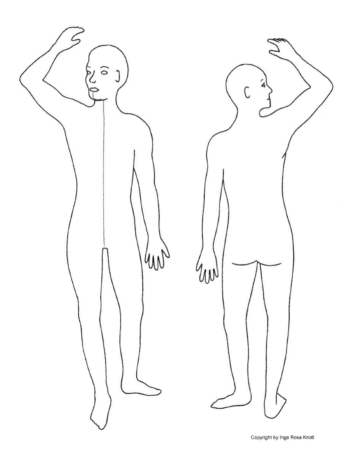

Copyright by Inge Rosa Knott

List of Energy Release Points for the Extraordinary Energy Release Channel of the Divine Feminine Matrix

Extraordinary Energy Release Channel of the Divine Masculine Director

The Energy Release Channel of the Divine Masculine Director is the aspect of the Divine Masculine Energy within the Creative Force, which is responsible for co-creation of the physical. It is partnered with the Divine Feminine Energy and work together for creation. If the Divine Feminine generates the potentials, it is the Divine Masculine that puts these potentials into motion. It is the action. It travels in a counter clockwise energetic pattern of direction. It creates and guides all communication that enables all the energy bodies, in all aspects and all directions, to work together in unified purpose. It is the inner vitality that draws on the resources from the movement of Spirit and its connection to Source. Connection to the Divine Masculine strengthens the energy of Divine Will with the flexibility of Cosmic Love.

Disharmonies: *Issues relating to survival and poverty consciousness; inability to flow with life; disconnection to spirit; over-striving beyond physical limits; fatigue; inner conflict with reconciling the material with spiritual existence; lack of integrity; inability to act on creative impulses. Physical manifestations of lower back pain; headaches; neurological disorders; poor memory.*

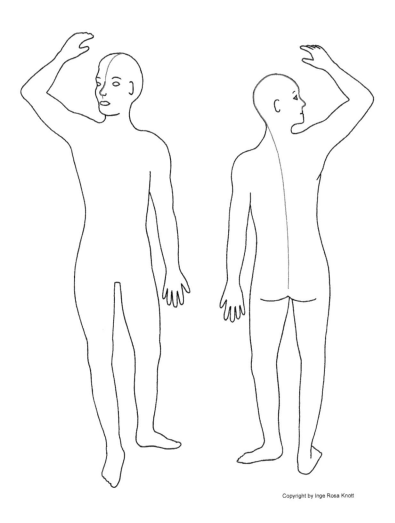

List of Energy Release Points for the Extraordinary Energy Release Channel of the Divine Masculine Director

Extraordinary Energy Release
Channel of the Penetrating Interface

The Extraordinary Energy Release Channel of the Penetrating Interface is the bridge between Heaven and Earth as manifested in humanity. It circulates energy up and down and strengthens our connection to our core identity and Divine Blueprint. It integrates the feminine and masculine vertical energy fields and is an interface between the Eight Extraordinary Energy Release Channels and the Twelve Energy Release Channels. It facilitates cosmic light, to penetrate into the depths of density, and retrieve the jewels hidden deep within. It penetrates into that which is dark, and through transformative alchemy, brings vitality to the Essence. It connects to initial patterns of life and assists in breaking through wounded intergenerational patterns for healing, renewal and re-birth. This Extraordinary Energy Release Channel is an interface between the masculine cosmic fire of creation, the feminine primordial water and the physicality of the Being. It is responsible for communicating the vitality of the Creative Force into the full body systems via the complete system of the Energy Release Channels. It is a vitality that moves our Essence and brings nourishment to all aspects of life. It creates and perpetually renews the pattern of life for each individual life stream.

Disharmonies: *Intergenerational cycles of disharmonies (physical, emotional, mental and spiritual); patterns of abuse and/or addictions; conscious or unconscious repetitive negative patterns of behaviour; intimacy issues; unresolved traumatic experiences; inability to manifest ideas. Physical manifestation of reproductive dis-orders; digestive disorders; eating disorders; pain in the chest; heart palpitations; oppression in the heart.*

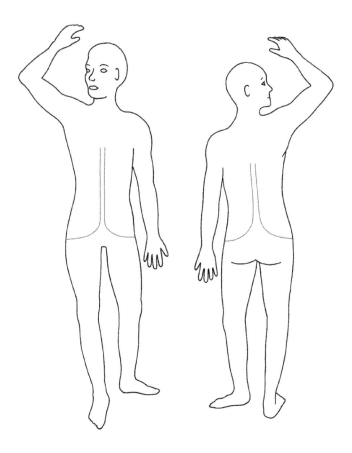

List of Energy Release Points for the Extraordinary Energy Release Channel of the Penetrating Interface

Extraordinary Energy Release Channel of the Vessel of Guidance

The Extraordinary Energy Release Channel of the Vessel of Guidance assists with the breaking of old patterns in order to further Soul evolution. It helps with rebuilding healthy ways of living in order to affirm and trust in the body's ability to self-heal, as well as optimize the reception of inspiration. The Vessel of Guidance connects to the horizontal energy field, communicating the blueprint of our body to our physical vehicle. It creates a structure of support. In this capacity, it harmonizes and creates a framework of structure to carry out Divine directives in the fulfillment of purpose. It is the only Extraordinary Energy Release Channel which flows horizontally. It is like a belt which gathers the directive power of the Extraordinary Energy Release Channel of the Divine Masculine Director (Governing Vessel), the creative power of the Extraordinary Energy Release Channel of the Divine Feminine Matrix (Conception Vessel) and the Divine blueprint of the Extraordinary Energy Release Channel of the Penetrating Interface (Penetrating Vessel). In this way, the Vessel of Guidance can circulate, strengthen and guide the energies for the implementation of rhythmic forward motion that is necessary in order to walk the path. It synchronizes communication and connections so that one can move life into action, from the strength of alignment, to the highest good of the One and of the ALL.

Disharmonies: *Frustration; procrastination; inability to find creative solutions and clear obstacles; stuck in old patterns of behaviour; inability to follow through on intentions; fence sitting; inertia; inability to evolve spiritually or conversely experience psychic imbalances from over expansion of spiritual forces. Physical manifestations of headaches; difficulty in urination; vaginal discharges; cold legs and feet; weakness or atrophy in the lower limbs; hip pain; sciatica.*

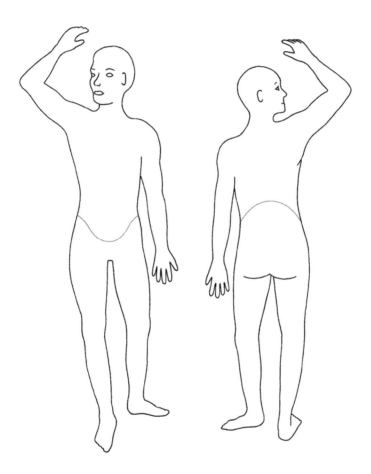

List of Energy Release Points for the Extraordinary Release Channel of the Vessel of Guidance

Extraordinary Energy Release Channel of the Feminine Vessel of Movement

The Extraordinary Energy Release Channel of the Feminine Vessel of Movement draws up vital strengthening creative energy from the watery depths of the Earth. It empowers illumination to comprehend the higher aspects of one's incarnation in relation to living a purposeful life. It creates the environment of internal reflection so that perception and focus are enhanced to support clarity of Soul vision. It ensures alignment with inner authenticity and Divine truths by strengthening core integrity, balance and centre through the connection with the stability of the Earth. The Feminine Vessel of Movement provides energy through consciousness which makes Ascension possible. It aligns with Divine Will and shines the light of illumination so that the Soul Essence can communicate clarity and focus, to being and living our purpose.

Disharmonies: *Anxiety; disconnection from Source; lack of clarity of purpose; inability to conceive or understand "why am I here?" "what is my purpose?"; lack of commitment; fear of transformational changes; inability to receive soul messages; lack of attunement; inability to see the bigger picture; depression; isolation; introversion. Physical manifestation of dry eyes; deteriorating vision; insomnia; muscle imbalances in the legs; abdominal distention; abdominal masses; equilibrium problems; structural imbalance between the left and right sides of the body such as in Parkinson's, MS or ALS; inability to feel the floor; feeling as though walking on a slant.*

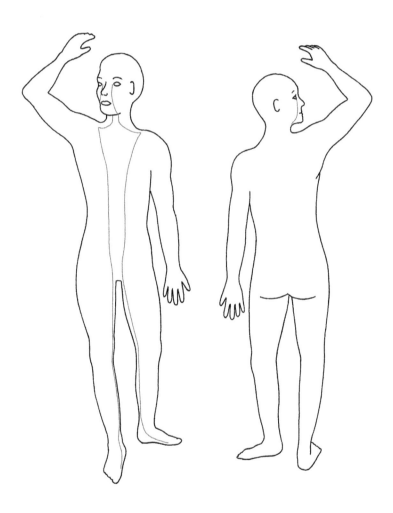

List of Energy Release Points for the Extraordinary Energy Release Channel of the Feminine Vessel of Movement

Extraordinary Energy Release Channel of the Masculine Vessel of Movement

The Extraordinary Energy Release Channel of the Masculine Vessel of Movement draws up energy from the heel of the foot in order to help one stand in a strong and erect manner. It harmonizes with the Extraordinary Energy Release Channel of the Feminine Vessel of Movement to assure the dynamic flow of energy drawn up from the depths of the Earth. It serves then to bring this Earth energy and direct it upwards to connect with the energy of Heaven and then circulate it through the body so that one successfully accomplishes one's mission. When connecting to this energy, one can visualize a mountain. The metaphor here is to connection with the strength of the mountain, its stability and rootedness. Its top piercing the clouds and connecting with the Cosmos. The body is a mountain. There is the reminder that our divinity is everlasting, that our Soul is immortal and we are here to ascend.

Disharmonies: *Nervous tension; easily overwhelmed by new information; control issues; inability to connect with intuition and insight; repetitive thoughts; chattering mind. Physical manifestations of severe dizziness; facial paralysis; deteriorating vision; stiff neck; hip pain; structural imbalances between the left and right sides of the body; problems with balance and equilibrium.*

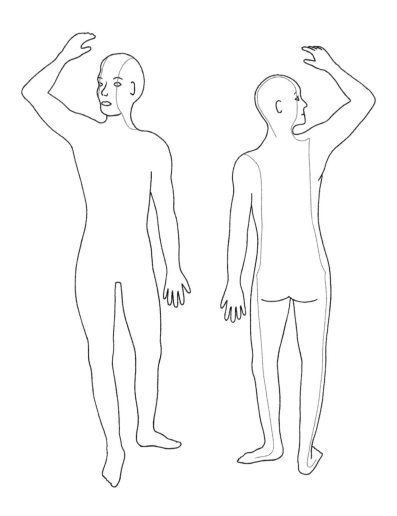

List of Energy Release Points for the Extraordinary Release Channel of the Masculine Vessel of Movement

Extraordinary Energy Release Channel of the Feminine Vessel of Structure

The Extraordinary Energy Release Channel of Structure provides connecting structures to link various aspects of the body together. When these links are established, the communication and cooperative forces are enhanced between all the Energy Release Channels as well as the organs, muscles and tissues of the physical body. They harmonize in joyful connectivity. This is a flexible network that allows for flowing receptivity and exchange, strengthening the ability to unwrap the heart with gratitude and to experience the feeling life of unconditional love. It is the embodiment of water. It symbolizes the power and wisdom of the mysterious feminine structure that permits us to ride the waves of life experience and work through difficult situations with ease and grace.

Disharmonies: *Feeling trapped; feeling powerless; anxiety; mental restlessness; depression; nightmares; flatness; inability to stay grounded; not in the body; paranoid; blame issues; inability to trust; emotionally shut down; intimacy issues; inability to give or receive love; depression. Physical manifestations of insomnia; chest pain; tightness in the chest; heart palpitations; pain at the back of the neck and occiput.*

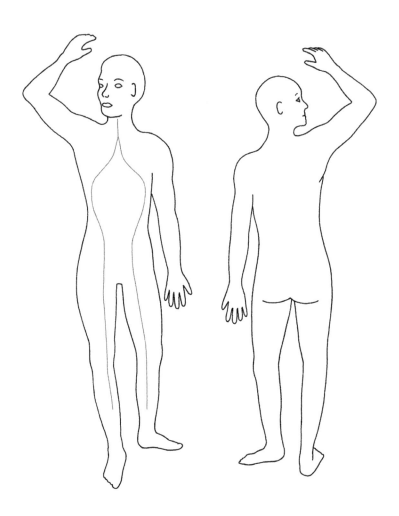

List of Energy Release Points for the Extraordinary Energy Release Channel of the Feminine Vessel of Structure

Energy Release Channel of the Masculine Vessel of Structure

The Extraordinary Energy Release Channel of the Masculine Vessel of Structure provides stability with the masculine energy. It empowers the health of the physical body and keeps everything in balance. It is an immune system interface which communicates between the environment of the inner physical body and that of the environment outside of the physical body. It assures that appropriate immune responses are activated. It is a strong defender that keeps all in harmony. It increases life energy so that one can encounter situations with confidence. It assists in balancing one's unique individuality, with the energy of group consciousness, so that one can function in wholeness within a larger social matrix.

Disharmonies: *Lack of confidence; dysfunctional in group settings; easily susceptible to external social demands; inability to connect to one's inner knowing; indecision; inability to let go of the past; fear of failure; being caught in a cycle of inaction; resentful or bitter in regards to authority figures and/or family; anger. Physical manifestations of low vitality; compromised immune system; shifting symptoms in disease patterns; pain in the lateral aspect of the legs; tinnitus; deafness.*

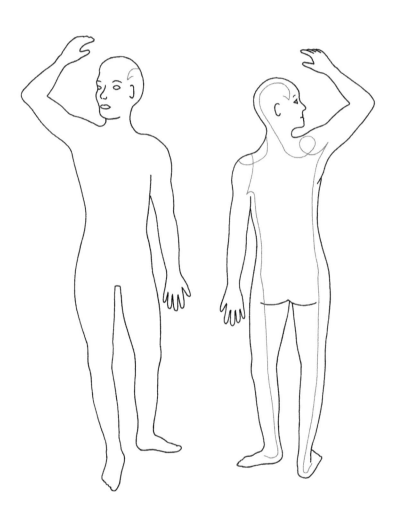

List of Energy Release Points for the Extraordinary Energy Release Channel of the Masculine Vessel of Structure

SECTION 3

Spiritual Portraits of the
Energy Release Points

Portraits of the Energy Release Points for the Energy Release Channel of the Lung

LU-1 Central Treasury

Virtues: This Energy Release point serves to empower inspiration and connection to Essence (Source) so that we are propelled toward our goals. It assists in helping us recognize and gain wisdom from our present life experience, our experiences in the earlier parts of our life as well as having compassionate understanding of our ancestry. When the revelations present, we are far more easily able to integrate these wisdoms with our present reality. Unblocking and activating this Energy Release Point allows for the process of self realization and the ability to make available our highest wisdom for conscious living in the present.

Disharmonies: *Loss of touch with our inner drive; lack of inspiration; internal emptiness; loneliness; blame issues.*

LU- 2 Cloud Gate

Virtues: This Energy Release Point clears grief that clouds the Heart so that we may more easily connect with the causes of emotional pain. Once the source of pain is identified, the ability to alchemically transform painful emotions into those of fulfillment and wholeness is strengthened. It empowers the ability to graciously accept and receive inspiration from the Universal All (Creative Force) as well as be receptive to the wisdom of others. It assists in the development of positivity and optimism so that one is empowered by reconnection to Soul vision. When unblocking and activating this Energy Release Point, it is helpful to visualize a heavenly light connecting through the upper energy centres into the brain/mind to unify with the light within the Heart. This being done, allow for the opening of the Heart to hope, to gratitude and to connection with the higher frequency of joy. This action of connecting and unifying the inspiration born of heaven within the Heart shows that this Energy Release Point has the additional function of being a gate. A well maintained gate opens with ease to welcome inspiration, hope and joy as guests and can close firmly to unwelcome guests such as negativity.

Disharmonies: *Chronic presence of grief, which can physically manifest as phlegm in the lungs; chronic cough and constant clear sinus dripping. (Symbolic representation of internal tears). Feeling forsaken and forgotten; expectation and anticipation of loss; feelings of emptiness; inability to receive what is of the greatest value both internally and externally; chronic negativity.*

LU-3 Heavenly Palace

Functions as a Window to Heaven point.

Sacred Storekeeper of the Akashic Records

Virtues: This Energy Release Point is a sacred storekeeper of the Akashic Records: the library of the Soul's journey. It is like being able to take a glimpse through the window to Heaven. Unblocking and activation of this Energy Release Point empowers one to find within themselves the highest expression of Heavenly inspiration. The Storehouse of the Eternal God; Our Soul Source. This allows us to connect to inspiration born of intrinsic Self Worth. To feel and receive the memory imprint of Divine virtue and inner purity. This is the place of virtue and purity that is untouched by life events. It serves as a reminder that Heaven/Divine/Universe can only see and find the best in us, despite life events and circumstances. It assists in the understanding that Heavenly justice is based on truths, free of judgment and compromise and that Heavenly justice is the embodiment of unconditional love. From this place of unconditional love, this Energy Release Point provides four important truths: Firstly, it provides access to inspiration from the grounded depths of spiritual Self Worth. Secondly, it cultivates the ability to forgive and to release emotional pain from the past so that one may move forward with freedom unburdened from life events. Thirdly, this Energy Release Point builds respect for self and for others as one begins to acknowledge the best within oneself and in others. Lastly, it allows for the internalization and integration of the relationship with Spirit; by connecting to the Divine it allows one to trust the inner teacher.

Disharmonies: *Compromise of value;, compromise of self; compromise of what is in the best interest of one's Soul or highest good; criticism; self judgment; judgment of others; finding and seeing only the worst of oneself or of others; perfectionism and disdain of what is less than perfect in oneself or others; unforgiving; bitter; holding onto pain and burdens from the past; disrespect; overly dependent on the external relationship to Spirit as personified by a spiritual teacher and institutions; hypocrisy developing from Disciple/ Teacher relationship.*

LU-4 Valiant White

Virtues: This Energy Release Point connects to the Ray of Divine Will. It guards and protects the spiritual flow of energy from the Source to our physicality. It brings purity of intention, courage, faith, initiative and dependability in regards to integrating one's will with the Divine Will. Unblocking and activating this Energy Release Point serves to raise our consciousness to the purity of intentions as inspired by Christ Consciousness (Unconditional Love). With this heightened consciousness, the development of Spiritual Warrior qualities are sparked from within and adds inner strength to act on inspiration.

Disharmonies: *Self righteousness; fanaticism.*

LU-5 Foot Marsh / Ghost Reception / Ghost Hall

Virtues: This Energy Release Point creates and strengthens a boundary that defines what is the Self and what is not. The strength of this boundary is determined by ones ability to discern and listen to what is of the highest good and in the best interest of the individual as well as acting upon the inner promptings. Unblocking and activating this Energy Release Point strengthens the connection to the inner truth of the Self. It helps one to recognize and remove oneself from situations in which one senses lower vibrational darker energies. In addition, activating this point will also release the energy of a possession (entity invasion, thought form, energy field invasion due to leaky aura). This speaks to its function as a ghost point as its name also implies.

Disharmonies: *Suffering and punishment; limiting belief systems in regards to sin, tribulation and suffering.*

LU-6 Greatest Hole

Virtues: This Energy Release Point creates movement allowing for the release of oppressed grief and longing. Grief that has been unexpressed, therefore stifled and repressed. This momentum of movement also releases the illusion that one is disconnected from life and the world around them. Once this movement begins to flow, it becomes easier for one to rediscover and connect with the pulse of life. As one unblocks this point the flow of release is enhanced by the visioning of a stream of tears flowing to an abyss or a great hole. Once grief has flowed through, this Energy Release Point empowers the virtue of emptiness so that we may transcend our sorrows and the pain of our little self, and by consequence, better appreciate and receive the value of what is present in each moment: joy, inspiration and lightness of being.

Disharmonies: *Sadness; longing; grief; overly sensitive; resignation; sorrow; holding on to memories and longing for old loves, friends, objects; attachments to the past.*

LU-7 Broken Sequence

Virtues: This Energy Release Point empowers the function of receiving inner clarity and letting go; surrendering that which no longer serves. It speaks to the Universal Principle that All is Rhythm. We receive and let go. We take in and we move out; everything is rhythmic and everything has an ebb and flow. When we seek to control or stop the rhythm, the sequence or Divine order of things seems broken and chaos ensues.

Unblocking and activating this Energy Release Point activates a return to balance by strengthening clarity of the concept of detachment and finding centre.

Disharmonies: *Lack of clarity; feelings of loss and longing stemming from childhood; difficulty with letting go and moving forward. Physical imbalances can manifest as things interrupted or out of rhythm: menstrual cycles, sleep cycles, eating disorders.*

LU-8 Energy Release Channel Gutter

Virtues: This Energy Release Point allows for the reception of purification and its processes that catalyze the alchemy to transcend and release what is called "mind over matter". One must release "mind over matter" and respect the needs of the body so that the whole being can connect to Essence. It assists in the ascension process of bringing the body along so that Heaven is created in the world of matter as a state of living in a higher frequency. Self Worth is empowered from the alignment of acting and living out inspiration. The ability of seeing ourselves as part of the weaving in the bigger picture is enhanced; to know that we are part of the manifestation of creation; the tapestry of life.   During European middle ages, historical events were woven into picture stories on the tapestries and entire histories of civilization are immortalized. Likewise, our individual thread, our lifestream creates a history; a story which connects us to our lineage of the past and to the formation and creation of the present and possible future. Life then becomes a series of events which we pass through. Unblocking and activating this Energy Release Point imparts the ability to connect to the value of past experience. It helps one to discern and allow the release of what is extraneous and not of value. This purification process allows for a cleansing and renewal in all aspects of Being. Through this process we may shine our essential selves to the world as an example of a life lived that is filled with inspiration and joy.

Disharmonies: *Congestion of the mind leading to congestion in the body - notably the sinus; depression; grief expressing as the body weeping - such as diarrhea.*

LU-9 Great Abyss / Great Spring / Ghost Heart

Virtues: This Energy Release Point inspires the movement of creation and connects one to the place between Heaven and Earth. The place where ideas are formed. It brings one back to The Origin, the source of all creation. It connects one to the Universal Principle that ALL is rhythm, and by so doing, empowers rhythmic movement in our Being. We are a reflection of the macrocosm; the rhythmic pulse of the Universe. Through this connection, the ability to feel gratitude and abundance is strengthened. As one connects with joy, one realizes that Heaven is a state of vibration within our perception and therefore, our source of nourishment and light for the Body and the Soul. Unblocking and activating this Energy Release Point opens us to the miracle of the gift of conception - of life itself. Father is viewed as Heaven giving the Soul Essence inspiration and luminosity. Mother is viewed as Earth nourishing the body through food and nutrients. These elements of both Father/Mother/Creative Force unite and integrate in each and every "now" moment. As the name Ghost Heart, this Energy Release Point releases possessive energies by surrendering all that is impure into the VOID while restoring our connection to our authentic self.

Disharmonies: *Materialism and greed; emptiness; loneliness; self isolation; depression; cravings for food, stimulants or material possessions; vacancy in the heart; joylessness; resignation; hopelessness.*

LU-10 Fish Region

Virtues: The name of this Energy Release Point is very symbolic of the Piscean Age where the symbol for God is the Fish. There are many references of fish in the New Testament of the Christian Bible - Master Jesus feeding the masses with fish; his followers being fishermen and transforming into "fishers of men" for example. The birthing place and dwelling of fish is water - vast oceans and seas. Symbolic of the water of Essence- the womb of Souls. Fish metaphorically become the representation of Source, which feeds us with Heavenly energy. This energy is pure fiery Essence. It is a fire greater than any fire known. The Alchemy is the transformational union of fire with the watery depths, bringing forth a completely new form by it's transformational properties. Unblocking and activating this Energy Release Point breaks us free from stagnation, inertia and emotional coldness by reconnecting our hearts to the Divine Heart. We are thus inspired to find the highest within ourselves so that we may move forward with empowered Self Worth, compassion and purpose.

Disharmonies: *Judgmental attitude towards self and others; low self esteem; self criticism; feelings of unworthiness; religious fanaticism; hard-heartedness.*

LU-11 Ghost Truth

Virtues: This Energy Release Point assists in balancing and regulating the connection between our vision of destiny and our ability to persevere towards the achievement of our goals. It helps to distinguish between selfless service and servitude. Discernment of the value of things; knowing when to conserve them and when to let them go. The realization that it is essential to let go versus the cost of holding on. Through this process we develop an understanding that constant feeding of the inessential drains and fractures the beautiful crystal structure of our Light Body. Unblocking and activating this Energy Release Point strengthens the ability to release what doesn't serve. Furthermore, vision and clarity in understanding of Self Worth is enhanced so that the Essential Self is valued as a priceless treasure.

Disharmonies: *Fractured consciousness; overwhelm leading to entity invasion and possession; always feeling or being caught in crisis situations.*

Portraits of the Energy Release Points for the Energy Release Channel of the Large Intestine

LI-1 Brilliant Exchange

Virtues: This Energy Release Point is the first in the series of the Energy Release Channel of the Large Intestine. As such, it is a point of entering or merging. It is a point of exiting the Spirit world and entering into Life in the Physical world. The movement from the Lung Energy Release Channel, inspiration of Spirit through breath, travels through the physical body to experience physical reality and finally, empowers the ability to receive pure intentional inspiration. One can then aspire and transcend the mundane and let go of what is not essential for the journey. It is similar to a brilliant merchant who can see the value of Essence and let go of all that does not correspond to the True Self. Unblocking and activating this Energy Release Point empowers the guarding of Soul virtue as treasure. It is a transformational point. One that brings awareness to the consciousness that the Soul has freely and lovingly exchanged it's heavenly experience for the experience of physical density and material existence. It is appropriate that this Energy Release Point was sounded into existence with the perfect fifth musical interval. The fifth is considered a jump off point - a musical space in which anything can manifest. This is a creative opening into an exciting new adventure likened to a composer's melodious creation. Transformation through which one purposefully leaps forward - empowered by the radiance and brilliance of light-filled clarity.

Disharmonies: *Hesitation; low self-esteem; self effacement; fear.*

LI-2 Between Two, the Second Interval

Virtues: This Energy Release Point describes the condition of being in the space or condition of a parenthesis, an interlude or interval. An interlude is a pause. An interval is a measure of space between two realities, two things or two sounds. It implies the space and moment in time of being between two conditions. These two conditions can be the completion of a step or phase of life and the next new venture or phase - that which is unknowable. In terms of the physical body it can be used to describe the transmission of a condition of dis-ease or disharmony from one organ to another. On the emotional and mental planes, it is the space within two states of being. On the spiritual plane, it is the state of duality, duplication and pause for reflection. Duality must exist in order for one to choose wholeness. Wholeness is achieved in the embracement of opposing poles. That is, to acknowledge the old lower painful aspects, integrate them through healing grace and thereby actively transform them. The release of the old creates the space for new higher vibrational experiences, such as joy, to manifest. Unblocking and activating this Energy Release Point provides calm within the process of the parenthesis. It empowers optimistic forward motion towards the unknown experiences yet to come.

Disharmonies: *To come from a place of vindictiveness; to drive a wedge between oneself and others or between oneself and one's goals; inability to create lasting friendships; polarization; to create obstacles and self sabotage; inability to forgive; judgmental attitude; inability to let go of the old.*

LI- 3 Small Valley, Third Interval

Virtues: This Energy Release Point is the metaphor of the third. It is the space between Heaven, Earth and Humanity. The number three is the creation of life between heaven and earth. It is the manifestation of the incarnated being. It speaks of the trinity and can be seen as the grandparent - child - grandchild. A representative of three generations. In the creation cycle of the five alchemical phases, wood is the grandchild of metal. In this new person, the grandchild, there is new creation. Here we find the new growth within ourself much like in the spring of the valley which comes to life with new creative processes. As the wood point of the Energy Release Channel of the Large Intestine, it brings the energy of growth. A renewal of inspiration, which comes from the release of what needed to be let go. Within the process of letting go, optimistic vision of the future, which is in harmony with the Divine Plan, ensures positive benevolent outcomes in alignment to internal truths and empowered self worth. Unblocking and activating this Energy Release Point allows for the interval, the interlude or space that one needs to integrate and process life events and learning lessons. The ability to release and receive a new perspective. It brings childlike innocence and trust in a benevolent and optimistic future as well as it assists one in staying in present time with wonder-filled appreciation and awe of the beauty of life.

Disharmonies: *Judgement; fanaticism; self-blame; feeling tainted by the past; low self-worth, inability to forgive.*

LI-4 Joining of the Valleys

Virtues: This Energy Release Point is an entrance way to amplified energized vitality. This vitality moves energy in order to let go of impurities, distortions, illusions, contamination and toxicity on all levels of the physical, emotional, mental and spiritual bodies. This amplification process is enabled through the power of unification. Valleys are deep, low lying areas surrounded by hills and/or majestic mountains. They are lush places of creation and growth, having ample water flow. Valleys are full of life. Joining of the Valleys represent the unification of more than one valley thus increasing it's potential in an infinite way. It can be visualized as rushing water, quickly flowing streams and rivers. It empowers receptivity to life and the courage to go forward, bringing untapped reserves of energy with unlimited potential. Unblocking and activating this Energy Release Point strengthens the commitment to oneself to end personal suffering as well as to release the attachment to suffering. This conscious act of connection to higher choice, higher awareness and higher vibration brings harmony to the whole body systems as well as the sensory systems. Once harmony is restored, the ability to access the inner chambers of the heart, where inner codes of cosmic star wisdom reside, can be facilitated with more ease.

Disharmonies: *Self destructive patterns; cycles of abuse; anxiety and fear; distress; stuck in victimization.*

LI-5 Stream of Masculine Energy

Virtues: This Energy Release Point balances inner conflict between the negative and positive ego. The ego strives to balance the ability to emanate power and often can be caught in a battle of wills when engaging with others. Unblocking and activating this Energy Release Point connects us to our inner light, helping us to feel great self love, self worth, and empowerment. There is a clear understanding of our Solar Self, our actions and our perceptions of truth. Understanding our unique individuality and the sacredness of the Divine Flame within, is key to Soul expression. From this understanding, one strengthens the ability to build a field that shields and protects while radiating our gifts from a place of balance and harmony. Nothing to prove, nothing to fear, nothing to try to control or to control in others. It is to be of service to the world in a selfless way, empowering the virtue of compassion.

Disharmonies: *Indiscrimination; overstepping boundaries; inner conflict; intolerance; self-righteousness; easily slighted leading to cold heartedness; obsessiveness; manias; bitterness; fear of losing control; fear of letting go of people; obsessive compulsive behaviours; worthlessness.*

LI-6 Side Passage

Virtues: This Energy Release Point can be visualized as a side passage or a side connection that interfaces with the Energy Release Channel of the Lung. The lung empowers the movement of Spirit, inspiration, freshness and life. The energetics of the lung is to receive heavenly inspiration for advancement of the life journey as directed by the Soul Essence. The energetics of the large intestine is to release the extraneous, so that forward fluid motion continues. Unblocking and activating this Energy Release Point strengthens the ability to receive and to let go, in a necessary and natural way. It means to allow the movement through Divine inspiration to a place of calm, where we are guided to let go of what is no longer of benefit. It removes stagnation caused by internalized grief and brings support in times of transition and change.

Disharmonies: *Feelings of being stuck, especially after a loss; unresolved grief.*

LI-7 Benevolent Warmth

Virtues: This Energy Release Point empowers the ability to release preconceived notions and judgments that block the ability to trust in the goodness of others. When there is trust, one can cultivate a flowing warmth of benevolence towards others. Unblocking and activating this Energy Release Point helps one to become warm and personable. It strengthens the knowing that in letting go of past hurts one is allowed a deeper exploration of the feeling life of the emotional body. This Energy Release Point helps to connect with the virtues of gratitude and compassion in regards to past experiences, thereby allowing for the receptivity of warmth to flow gentle benevolence. In this way, the conditions required for creating a positive and optimistic future are supported.

Disharmonies: *Cold within the physical, emotional and mental bodies; inflexibility; tendency to perfectionism; self-righteousness; attitude of distaste and aloofness; rigidity of mind; disdain of others; persecution complex; insecure in relationships; social barriers.*

LI-8 Lower Side

Virtues: This Energy Release Point brings strength and stability to our core, the place of centre where we find balance and harmony, movement and flexibility. It is to stand on the solid ground and stability of earth. From this support, we can develop our skills, cultivate our knowledge, strengthen our integrity and strive towards mastery in our craft. Unblocking and activating this Energy Release Point strengthens our centre. It helps with the assimilation, digestion and integration of life experiences and allows for the flow of movement through the release of negativity.

Disharmonies: *Experiencing periods of stagnation and apathy; negativity.*

LI- 9 Upper Integrity

Virtues: This Energy Release Point brings the impetus to rise to the highest and best of who we are in order to walk our path to the best of our ability. It is growth from our centred self to the highest level of integrity, impeccability, enthusiasm and joyous expression of our creative selfs. Unblocking and activating this Energy Release Point allows for the drawing in and receptivity of heavenly inspiration. It frees the flow of spontaneity that comes from a place of unwavering trust in the Divine Plan. We recognize our place within the plan, and trust in the attainment of the most benevolent outcome. The ability to eliminate waste and to assimilate and digest positive life experiences is enhanced thus restoring vitality, enthusiasm and motivation for doing and serving others.

Disharmonies: *Holding on to what has no value to avoid the grief of loss; digestive disorders; physical weakness in the arms.*

LI-10 Arm Three Measures / Ghost Evil

Virtues: This Energy Release Point speaks to the ability to cross the distance, to make the necessary steps to approach and deliver one's message. It helps one to walk firmly on the Earth, arms outstretched to the cosmos, so that one can receive inspiration, strength and support. The number three in the name, Arm Three Measures, signifies the union of the three flowing energies. Firstly, to connect with the Universal Mind. Secondly, to flow inspiration from the Universal Mind to the Intellectual Mind. Lastly, to walk purposefully in grounded steps, the path of a fulfilled Soul directed life. The alternate name, Ghost Evil, speaks to the myriad of distractions that present along the journey which circumvent our ability to express our truth and deliver our message. Unblocking and activating this Energy Release Point allows for a connection between the Point of Light within the Universal Mind to that of the individual Intellectual Mind. Furthermore, it empowers a flowing conduit towards physical action as it facilitates the ability to come out of the mind and intellect to create viable action. It empowers the ability to extend oneself to active participation in life and social involvement through meaningful activity.

Disharmonies: *Intellectual exhaustion; pain in the physical arm when extending outwards; inability to express and deliver one's message; inability to take viable action towards living purposefully; lack of stamina; lack of strength; lack of vitality; obsessive attachment to accumulation of material wealth; exhaustion and fatigue; inability to reap rewards of work well done or joy in life.*

LI-11 Crooked Pond / Ghost Minister

Virtues: This Energy Release Point brings nourishment, strength, security, balance, and stability through the reconnection to Divine Mother consciousness as well as Earth Mother energies. Unblocking and activating this Energy Release Point actively brings one to the state of being held securely in the arms of a mother. A place of safety, warmth and calm. This is especially important as one works through the understanding of Karma - to look at the bigger picture of events, learn the required lesson and invoke forgiveness. Connecting to the Divine Mother and asking for Divine Grace cleanses the body systems of fear and allows for the release of karmic lessons while keeping the jewels of wisdom. Connecting to the Earth Mother strengthens the ability to draw the nutrients from our sources of food in order to be enriched, cared for and nurtured. The ability to intake food and life experiences, digest and process them, restores the balance between intake and elimination. As the alternate name suggests, this Energy Release Point assists in exorcising ghosts from the past, releasing them so that one feels the impetus of forward movement.

Disharmonies: *Emptiness; loneliness; abandonment; inability to let go of the past; failure to move forward; no conscious recognition of the Universal Law of Cause and Effect and karmic patterns; stagnation; distress; anxiety; depression; feelings of being out of control; auto-immune disorders; physical manifestation of hives.*

LI-12 Elbow Crevice

Virtues: This Energy Release Point speaks to the ability to release the extraneous or superfluous material which blocks discernment and mental clarity. Many times, that which is extra or unpleasant is put away in a hidden place - a closet, a box, or a crevice. Not wanting to throw it away, yet not knowing what to do with it. This is regardless of whether it is material or emotional in nature, hence the expression "out of sight, out of mind". However, after the passage of time, accumulation builds and things can leak, seep or ooze out of corners, closets or crevices. One is then faced with the daunting task of peeling through the layers, sifting through and cleaning up. This in itself can lead to more overwhelm or fatigue; the end result being indiscriminate purging just to get it over with. This Energy Release Point keeps things in balance. It harmonizes the thinking forces so that one may deal with things in an appropriate manner as they present. It raises the level of order and discernment so that one may flow with the rhythm of life.

Disharmonies: *Paralysis and stagnation in the mind and body; physical pain in the elbow; inability to release the inessential and stretch arms to grasp the new or to embrace life. Physically one may experience digestive disorders such as irritable bowel syndrome.*

LI-13 Arm Five Miles / The Working Strength of Five

Virtues: This Energy Release Point speaks to the powerful strength that is available through honouring the flow and movement of the Universal Laws. The Fifth Universal Principle is the Law of Rhythm. This Universal Principle speaks to the power of being in centre in order to facilitate rising above the Law. Centre is the place from which all directions and endless potential possibilities flow. The understanding and application of this Universal Principle allows one to tap into great energy and movement and use this energy as resources for the building of stamina. The stamina required to make change. The Fifth Universal Principle states that ALL is Rhythm; everything flows. To receive in the hand, embrace and take action with the arm, then allow the flow of the outcome.

Disharmonies: *To have extreme opposites such as: to hold on tightly or to indiscriminately let everything go; to stagnate and be unable to take action or to be overactive leading to overwork and exhaustion.*

LI-14 Upper Arm

Virtues: This Energy Release Point connects us to the identity of our True Self and our inner authority as decreed by the Creative Force. In many organizations, the badge of authority is sewn on the upper arm of a jacket. This would be the illusion of outer authority, such as that of high ranking government or military officials, or identities of a cultural group such as the Jewish peoples in World War II. The True Self does not require outer identity or outward signs acknowledging its authority. The True Self has the knowledge and wisdom of the Creative Force through the Connection to the I AM Presence within. This connection ensures the guidance needed to direct one's life in purity, wisdom and heavenly justice. Unblocking and activating this Energy Release Point draws forth the vitality necessary to live a life of courage and authenticity. It empowers living our truth and moving forward in confidence, respect and dignity for self and for others.

Disharmonies: *Grief; longing; control issues especially around relationship; excessive pride; feelings of superiority; prejudice.*

LI-15 Shoulder Majesty

Virtues: This Energy Release Point addresses the ability to shoulder responsibility in a strong and capable manner. The name Shoulder Majesty invokes the image of dignity, strength, self empowerment, healthy self esteem and Mastery. A well run kingdom has the qualities of strong management and clarity, working for the benefit of the people. The shoulder is located between the mind and the heart and serves as intermediary. It integrates the clarity of what needs to be done with the forces of the heart, empowering compassion and love based service. It allows for clear discernment and strengthens the ability to respond to what is to be let go and what is to be retained. Unblocking and activating this Energy Release Point strengthens the ability to shoulder responsibility and release feelings of burden. It helps to extend oneself in heart-based service to humanity. It further empowers one to surrender, ask for, and accept the assistance of others when necessary.

Disharmonies: *Over-striving beyond one's limits leading to physical exhaustion; unyielding; inability to ask and/or receive help from others; martyrdom; continual rescuing behaviour; hero complex.*

LI-16 Great Bone

Virtues: This Energy Release Point has two important aspects within the name - the noun Bone and its adjective Great. Bones, in and of themselves, are the structure of the body. They are the foundation of where we have come from. Within the bones, are the memories of our experiences as well as those of our genetic lineage, flowing within the bone marrow. Our foundation and structure of the bones create the shape of our body. Within the foundation and structure of the bones - our bone marrow, genetic lineage, family, cultural traditions and our values, create the shape of our lives. Within all this is the Seed Memory of the gift of being created. The remembrance of the Great Soul Within. The Soul has great work to do. It is said that great work requires great intensity and Soul passion. This Energy Release Point calls us to our Mastery. Mastery assists in the release of that which blocks the cultivation of our gifts. It empowers the ability to stand tall, with dignity and healthy esteem born of our worthiness. In this way, the strength required to shoulder our responsibilities flow with ease from the foundation of our bones. Unblocking and activating this Energy Release Point reminds one of the greatness within, our worthiness and the realization of the importance of what we bring to the world.

Disharmonies: *Low self worth; feelings of unimportance; contempt; bitterness; overwhelmed by duties and responsibilities; structural aches in the shoulders and neck.*

LI-17 Heavenly Vessel or Heavenly Summit

Virtues: This Energy Release Point empowers the virtues of emptiness, openness and purity. Virtues which help to diminish the feelings of unworthiness and shame, as well as feelings of being tainted. Heavenly Vessel, in Taoism, evokes the image of a bronze vessel with three legs used in sacred ritual for offerings to heaven. The offering is sent up in prayer and in return, the aspirant receives spiritual influence and wisdom. The three legs symbolize the unity of Heaven, Humanity and Earth. This sacred vessel was also used in banquets to hold nourishment for the Emperor. In our modern time, the Emperor becomes a metaphor for the God within us. The I AM Presence. In order to connect to the I AM Presence, the conditions of existential emptiness and purity must be in place in order for it to be worthy to hold offerings and receive spirit. The ritual of emptying, cleaning, offering and receiving, represents the transition to a refined quality of Essence. This creates the sense of openness and purity, thereby releasing the separation between heart and mind. Unblocking and activating this Energy Release Point serves to align us with the highest of that which the Divine Self has placed within us. Through this alignment, the energy is in place to continually strive for enlightenment, illumination and Soul evolution towards Ascension.

Disharmonies: *Unworthiness; self effacement; self deprecation; shame.*

LI-18 Support and Rush Out

Virtues: This Energy Release Point can be visualized as a chimney, that when open, properly vents out smoke and regulates airflow. If the chimney has not been used properly or has not been well maintained, there can be a build up of soot and debris causing obstructions and congestion of the flow. The chimney in early dwellings of ancient times was usually found in the centre of the home. It provided not only structural support for the building but also provided a gathering place for family and community. It gave emotional and physical support through social interaction, the preparation and the eating of food, as well as providing warmth. Unblocking and activating this Energy Release Point allows us to evaluate our supports. It allows for an opening, similar to that of a window, through which built up congestion can rush out to restore proper flow. It brings clarity and enlightenment. This enlightenment is precisely the ability to see how holding on to what is not good for us, such as resentment, past hurts and grief prevent us from seeing our gifts and who we truly are. This insight inspires freshness of a new vision of the present and a vision of a positive, optimistic future. The world and life become more sacred. Support, enthusiasm and fresh creativity is enhanced to live more joyfully in the world.

Disharmonies: *Feeling unsupported by male figures, such as the father in childhood or the Divine; inability to let go of past grievances; inability to receive; lack of inspiration or enthusiasm; inability to harmonize breathing; clinging to the past due to grief of a great loss.*

LI-19 Grain Hole

Virtues: This Energy Release Point is an alchemical transformational point. It assists in the quality of discernment and refines what is essential and what is extraneous. This refinement process is similar to the flow of grain through the polishing mill to remove the chaff from the germ - the germ being the heart of the grain. This allows for the gathering of the beautiful germ within the grain, that is, to discern the quality of the jewel: the seed or the truth of our experiences. Unblocking and activating this Energy Release Point empowers wisdom from perspective and discernment. It allows us to gather, digest and integrate the messages of wisdom that we discern within the layers of life experiences as we release the extraneous to refine the learning.

Disharmonies: *Lack of discernment; overwhelmed by the bombardment of chaos.*

LI-20 Welcome Fragrance

Virtues: This Energy Release Point empowers the ability to embrace the wholeness of life. It brings clarity, positive outlook and mental alertness. It empowers receptivity and openness. Unblocking and activating this Energy Release Point brings us into present time, the place where we can fully appreciate the beauty and vibrancy of life. It clears the way, removes obstacles and allows us to be present in the face of opportunities so that we can continue to flow along our path with clarity of direction, enabling a higher perspective and cosmic vision.

Disharmonies: *Failure to digest life; negativity; pessimism.*

Portraits of the Energy Release Points for the Energy Release Channel of the Stomach

ST-1 Receive Tears / Flowing Tears

Virtues: This Energy Release Point helps to flow emotional congestion in order to understand and receive insightful nourishment from painful experiences. The Soul experiences emotions through the interaction of the emotional body with the physical body. When painful emotions are experienced, there can be a detachment; a coping mechanism. This detachment serves to anesthetize the feeling life. Detachment over time can lead to a false mask of cheerfulness, denial, or addictive behaviours, which ultimately creates congestion in the physical body. This congestion can present not only as digestive issues but also cause body inflammation, particularly in the elimination system and in the sinus cavity. Unblocking and activating this Energy Release Point is similar to opening a floodgate which relieves and cleanses this emotional congestion. Once the congestion is released, it becomes easier to acknowledge and work with emotional pain, receive nourishment and understand the painful aspects of the past. With the re-establishment of flow and movement, reception of wisdom is facilitated as well as the ability to let go is enhanced. In this way, the Soul continues to learn and grow in wisdom and emotional strength.

Disharmonies: *Inability to cry; feeling heavy or oppressed; inability to let go of the past; needy behaviour; manipulation of others through tears.*

ST-2 Energy of Four Whites

Virtues: This Energy Release Point refers to the four white areas of the eye surrounding the iris as well as the purity of the Soul. It brings clarity of vision. It is said that the eyes are the windows to the Soul. The Soul has vision. A vision which is expansive, creative and filled with joyful desire. When this vision becomes obscured and loses its focus, one feels stagnant, devitalized and overwhelmed with the mundanity of daily living. The number four represents the movement of Spirit as it flows effortlessly like the winds in the four directions between Heaven, Earth and the Human. The number four is also a symbol of geometry as it is constructed of a triangle and a T-square; both very important instruments of the draftsman.

This suggests planning and order. Unblocking and activating this Energy Release Point allows the connection to the Soul's perfect memory to realize and express creative potential through the instrument of the physical body. It stimulates clarity of vision. It brightens the outlook towards positivity and assists one in formulating goals to achieve one's purpose. Energy of Four Whites empowers one to look beyond the mundane and find clear direction. It is through living our vision that one can more easily digest and receive nourishment from life. It strengthens the ability to extract the energy needed for purposeful action so that one proceeds with joyful enthusiasm for life and the world.

Disharmonies: *Inability to see and connect to one's Soul vision; physical manifestations of sore, tired, red eyes; fatigue and weariness; swelling in the eyes.*

ST-3 Great Hole

Virtues: This Energy Release Point addresses the ability to release excessive thought and worry in order to obtain inner peace. It is the ability to be emotionally honest with oneself, acknowledge emotional pain and remove the mask of cheerfulness used as a coping mechanism when facing the world. It accesses our inner core and provides the strength and courage to deal with the worries that deplete our vitality and compromise mental stability. The physical location of this Energy Release Point is in the hole of the cheek bone. Bones provide structure and protection for the whole body. Unblocking and activating this Energy Release Point brings connection to the inner core of the bones and the centre of one's Being where roots of security and stability are accessed. Strengthening the connection to the bones and centre of Self, strengthens the feelings of stability, security and protection. This flow of vital strength brings courage to the forefront to address emotional pain and the fortitude to continue despite obstacles in the navigation through life. Ultimately, one feels the freedom to live authentically, in positive vulnerability and Soul expression.

Disharmonies: *Worrisome thoughts; having a busy mind; denial and avoidance of emotional pain. Physical manifestations of pain and numbness of the face and lips; toothaches.*

ST-4 Earth Granary / Earth Greening

Virtues: This Energy Release Point harmonizes the relationships between appetite, need and nourishment. The name itself brings into our consciousness the image of our Earth and it's potential of being an unlimited source of nourishment. In the alternate name, the picture of Earth Greening speaks of abundance, health, vitality and fertility. Greening is the movement of transformative regenerated energy which is witnessed in the spring. Greening is the word used by the mystic St. Hildegard of Bingen to describe the breath of the Holy Spirit of God giving life to all things. A granary functions as a storage facility. It stores the reserves of nourishment from the harvest and symbolizes abundance and security. Unblocking and activating this Energy Release Point brings into our consciousness the remembrances of knowledge that all is provided. One has what is needed and now can be empowered to assist others. From this realization of abundance, true generosity and altruism are nourished. This Energy Release Point also speaks to our relationship with our mother as a physical embodiment of the greater "Earth Mother" or "Feminine Nurturing Matrix". Ideally, the balanced mother teaches and models for her infants and children, appropriate boundaries in life. Teaching through this balanced identification of herself, bringing the fulfillment of both her needs and the needs of the children. By extension, the needs of the entire family are met and hence assists with the interactions of the individual within the larger community.

Disharmonies: *Selfishness; habitual giving; hoarding tendencies; feelings of not having enough; neediness; inability to receive; disempowerment. Physical manifestations can present as anorexia; bulimia; binge eating; emotional eating; digestive issues; cravings especially for sweets.*

ST-5 Great Welcome

Virtues: This Energy Release Point helps us to see the wealth of our Essence and the unique gifts that only we can bring to the world. It is to know that we are welcomed by the world and earthly life, as well as to help us reciprocate and welcome the world. When one connects to their intrinsic self worth, dignity and self respect, the ability to receive and welcome life is empowered from within. It means to walk with dignity remaining open to the greatness of our potential. It inspires the virtue of flexibility in the face of curves and obstacles that the journey of life presents. The Soul becomes strong, resilient and vibrant. This strong Soul welcomes life and welcomes people, knowing it is safe, secure, warm and nourished. Unblocking and activating this Energy Release Point strengthens our centre with the perception of our gifts and empowers our self worth. Life and people are embraced and a deeper awareness of how one may develop and utilize their gifts to best serve the needs of others is enhanced.

Disharmonies: *Closed off to life; fear and negativity surrounding events; inability to trust in the goodness of others; tension in the jaw area from overthinking and "chewing over" words, events and actions; self doubt; resentment; avoidance of confrontation; bitterness; feeling "sour" manifesting physically as a sour taste in the mouth and/or acid reflux.*

ST-6 Jaw Vehicle / Motion Gate / Ghost Forest

Virtues: This Energy Release Point addresses the importance of the mouth: the jaw in particular and its role in the cycle of ingesting, digesting and flowing nurturance. It is part of the continuous circle of receiving nourishment, both from food and life experience, and actively transforming it for easier assimilation and digestion. The jaw bone becomes the vehicle of motion through which the action of chewing creates an environment conducive to swallowing food and life experience. It provides a space to chew over and evaluate how we give and receive, as well as provides the opportunity to recognize one's needs. Unblocking and activating this Energy Release Point helps us to acknowledge, chew over and quickly discern what are the essentials for balanced giving and receiving. It empowers clear, healthy expression of one's needs so that one can flow nurturance to self and to others. The alternate name, Ghost Forest, is in reference to this Energy Release Point as a ghost point. The name alludes to ghosts trapped within the darkness of the forest, emanating sounds of their torment borne on the wind. Unblocking and activating this Energy Release Point with the intention of releasing this trapped ghost energy, assists in releasing tension in the jaw. This allows for the release of stifled, deeply buried dark emotions. This release imparts the ability to confront and actively transform destructive emotions of the shadow side, integrating them into acceptance and light. Ghost Forest is also the Energy Release Point used to release clenched jaws during epileptic seizures which ancient cultures believed to be brought on by sudden invasion of ghosts.

Disharmonies: *Unbalanced relationship to nurturance; excessive chewing manifesting as worry and obsessive thought; excessive deliberation; inability to flow with life; haunted by past experiences resulting in difficulty carrying on and forward movement; physical manifestations of teeth grinding, TMJ and jaw tension.*

ST-7 Lower Passage of Earth

Virtues: This Energy Release Point is a gate opening to a passageway that descends deep into the Earth. It is about a strong rooted connection to grounding, stability and security. It is a place of connection to the Essence of Earth. A connection which brings nourishment and abundant resources available to us for sustenance and growth. This Energy Release Point also connects to other vital systems of the physical body, creating a network of supply so that the physical body stays balanced, nourished and vital. Unblocking and activating this Energy Release Point empowers the ability to ask for what one needs and lends strength to the connection to a centre of stability and abundance, thereby empowering giving and receiving.

Disharmonies: *Inability to receive; inability to give; fear of lack; tension in the jaw; frustration; disconnection from Earth; uprootedness; inability to stay centred and grounded.*

ST-8 Head Tied

Virtues: This Energy Release Point strengthens the ability to calm the mind and form logical, connected streams of thought out of chaotic, disconnected and churning thoughts. It helps break the pattern of cycles found within the chaos and disconnected thoughts when a mind obsessively repeats a loop of thinking. The pattern, once broken, allows for calm resolution of thought, creating order and harmony in the mind. Once this resolution takes place, the ability to detach from worry and connect to the truth and wisdom of the heart is facilitated. Centre, balance and calm allows for clarity of thought. Thought becomes empowered by intention. Unblocking and activating this Energy Release Point strengthens intentional integrity of thought by connecting the mind to the Wisdom of the Heart. The alignment of thought, speech and action empowers overall feelings of flow, balance and grounded centre. Physically, integrity can manifest as a healthy digestive system. A digestive system that not only has the ability to receive and integrate nourishment, but also has the ability to recognize and strengthen conscious eating. Knowing when enough is enough and recognizing when one is satisfied and content.

Disharmonies: *Worry; repetitive and obsessive thoughts; inability to process information; obsessive catering to one's own needs or the needs of others; imbalances in giving and receiving; overly sympathetic behaviour; inability to recognize boundaries where giving and doing for others undermines the ability to tend to one's own needs; chewing over the same thoughts while being unable to take productive action; continuous replaying of events and conversations in the mind; unconscious eating such as reading, watching television or a computer screen while eating; digestive disorders.*

ST-9 Welcoming Humanity as Part of All

Virtues: This Energy Release Point embodies the principle that "ALL is in the ALL" and "The ALL is in ALL". It is the unity of consciousness. The awareness that humanity is a part of nature, that nature is a part of Heaven, Earth and Humanity. Humanity, therefore, is the totality of the ALL. Connecting with this Energy Release Point connects us with our centre where we feel communion and belonging to the Earth. A sense of home, a sense of support, a unification with all that surrounds us. We feel connected and in union, and this feeling energizes and boosts vitality. Unblocking and activating this Energy Release Point provides the opening to receive and feel the great connection with the Universal ALL. A connection which brings great welcome and joyous connection to Essence. The connection with Essence clears and empowers vision and enables one to stand upright with dignity so that the ability to set appropriate boundaries regarding giving is empowered. It fuels Heart's desire to open, cultivate compassion, revive generosity of sharing and receiving so that life is filled with beauty and enriched with abundance. This Energy Release Point furthermore acts to help distinguish one's own needs from those of others, therefore releasing dysfunctional relationships and re-harmonizing to the Divine Feminine Mother who nourishes and supports in a healthy way.

Disharmonies: *Isolation; hardened heart; lack of joy; lack of love; lack of desire; feeling unsupported; disconnected from spirit; narrow scope of vision; paranoid; antagonistic projection; misperception of reality; inability to grow, change or move forward; inability to say no; resentment resulting from habitual giving; ingratiation; hiding our true intentions in order to avoid conflict; co-dependence; neediness.*

ST-10 Water Rushing Out / Water Gate / Water Heaven

Virtues: This Energy Release Point empowers verbal communication which is harmonized with the heart. It allows for speaking of what one needs from a place of love and emotional balance. Water represents Source as well as Primordial power and vitality. Connecting with this Energy

Release Point allows for lively expression. It helps to articulate dynamic speech which clearly defines healthy boundaries. Unblocking and activating this Energy Release Point assists in connecting with this dynamic energy in order to flow the ability of expression via the channel of the heart. In this way, expression harmonizes with the will and the ability to have a breakthrough in communication is enhanced. Words can be exchanged in a loving compassionate way, harmonizing relationships with people and with life.

Disharmonies: *Stagnation in throat and communication manifesting as physical blockages in the throat; inability to set boundaries in accordance to one's needs; tension in the throat and neck area; harsh and/or destructive communication; verbal aggression.*

ST-11 Spirit Cottage

Virtues: The Energy Release Channel of the Stomach is considered to correspond to the energy of Earth Mother and its qualities of nurturance, security and stability. This Energy Release Point, as well as the four which follow, have names which generally represent home elements which can be mundane yet comforting nonetheless. Beginning with Spirit moving from the lofty heavenly aspect of the world of Ether to ground into the physical body through the nurturing mother aspect, we see Spirit moving from the spiritual realms of glory, into the simplicity of the cottage. Spirit transforms itself from the point of Light within the mind of the Universal ALL to the point of Light within the mind of humanity. Movement from the realm of Palaces to the realm of mind/thought within the realm of the Cottage. The Cottage, in it's simplistic sense, is a place to live, to rest, to stop or to find shelter - much as the Earth itself is home to our humanity. It is a place where we embody in physicality and receive nourishment and comfort. Spirit Cottage is an Energy Release Point which balances and integrates the welcoming in of Spirit into the body. It nourishes both the physical and spiritual aspects of our being so that our mind creates and our actions manifest our creations from a heart, love and spiritual base. Therefore, our ability to fulfill our desires and find contentment, stability and peace throughout our life's journey is dependent upon the integrity of alignment of heart/mind (spirit/physical) and our ability to feel at home in wholeness and completeness in any circumstance or situation in which we find ourselves. Our outward life of centre, security and stability is a direct reflection of our ability to be comfortable, secure and centred within ourselves. This Energy Release Point nourishes communication between our minds and our hearts so that we feel secure and centred in all aspects of our Being.

Disharmonies: *Insecurity and anxiety due to childhood memories of instability or abandonment; feelings of displacement due to divorce or family breakdown; dislocation due to frequent moving or traveling; feelings of homelessness; inability to find and connect to community.*

ST-12 Broken Bowl

Virtues: This Energy Release Point assists in reconstructing that which is shattered. This shattering of the energy field and emotional body can occur when one experiences great loss and remains in illusion and victim consciousness. This state of emotional pain or shatter comes from having poured oneself so completely into another that the integrity of one's wholeness cannot withstand the void of emptiness. This can come from endings of dysfunctional, co-dependent relationships of all kinds. (Parent/child, husband/wife, romantic relationships, and friendships for example). Unblocking and activating this Energy Release Point assists in moving through grief and loss. It assists in raising the consciousness from a personal ego centre to a transcendent larger picture. Moving pain into the heart space to be transformed to peace, forgiveness and joy in order to release suffering and re-birth. This transformational point assists in detachment and viewing the larger perspective. To see transition and change as an opportunity for growth; growth filled with enthusiasm of the new life experience which awaits. It empowers emotional freedom and unconditional love so that Soul evolution can continue in a self-sufficient way.

Disharmonies: *Neediness; co-dependency; worry; drama filled relationships; empty nest syndrome; stage parent; control issues; intense grief; victim consciousness; personal attachment; loss of self; loss of individuality; inappropriate boundaries between parents and children. Physically this point impacts milk production for breast feeding, symbolizing self care; nurturance; teaching healthy boundaries to the baby; mother/child bonding. Improper bonding creates distrust of the world, instability of one's centre and growing into a dysfunctional adult; inability to provide for oneself the nourishment affecting the ability to be self sufficient. (Physically, mentally, emotionally and spiritually). In Broken bowl, life is shattered, the illusion is broken and one falls to pieces.*

ST-13 Door of Vital Nourishing Energy

Virtues: This Energy Release Point speaks to the virtue of being on a threshold that one is compelled to cross. The nature of a door is that it can open and close. When open one moves through easily, connecting and keeping a receptive state, trusting that support and compassion are available and easily integrated into one's awareness. When doors are flowing well, life flows well. Experiences provide opportunities for growth and the development of wisdom. Unblocking and activating this Energy Release Point strengthens the ability to draw on the vitality of life. It fuels the ability to flow with a flexible, open mind. It empowers one to embrace life in all its present moments while reciprocally receive nourishing vitality that living in wholeness offers.

Disharmonies: *Having difficulty accepting compassion and support; frustrated by the compulsion to transform or bring into fruition a passion or project due to fighting an "uphill battle"; inflexible mind; unwillingness to view things in a new way; fear of the unknown; fear of change; closing oneself off to participating in life.*

ST-14 Storehouse

Virtues: This Energy Release Point strengthens the ability to assimilate inspired directives of Spirit and integrate them through the physical vehicle of our body. Through the alchemical process of the elixir of Spirit and nourishment of the Divine Mother, one can more easily connect to stores of vitality and potentialize the fulfillment of purpose. It allows for the receipt of transformational experience that is in resonance with our essential Self and to fearlessly move through and release that which is not in resonance. It empowers the ability to see things as they are with objectivity and positive light in order to move through these experiences free from fear. It strengthens Soul's desire in such a way that we can fuel and fulfill our destiny. In this way, we may progress with Soul Evolution. Unblocking and activating this Energy Release Point empowers the unification of wisdom from the Divine Source of inspiration and our vitality in our physicality to fulfill our potential for our life purpose.

Disharmonies: *Dissatisfaction - always feeling hungry for something more; feeling unfulfilled; inability to connect with inspiration; lack of willpower; fatigue.*

ST-15 Feather Screened Room

Virtues: This Energy Release Point creates a space of peace where one feels protected and safe. This is especially important during times of intimate contact and sexual expression so that heartfelt love can flow unrestricted with positive vulnerability. Unblocking and activating this Energy Release Point allows for the gentle expression of intimacy, a sharing of the heart and an appreciation of the beauty found within the Self as well as within others.

Disharmonies: *Sensitivity to being seen; fear of intimate contact; history of sexual abuse.*

ST-16 The Window of the Breast

Virtues: This Energy Release Point encapsulates the vision of both nourishment and nurturance. It brings the experience of sacred love, security, stability and comfort. The Window of the Breast re-establishes connection to the energy of this experience. From this place, one can view and choose participation in life with renewed trust, knowing that one is held not only in the arms of the Divine Mother, but that one can also draw strength and nurturance from one's inner centre. It allows for the freedom to be curious and explore the world with the ability to know when to withdraw and replenish oneself with the loving care of feminine energy. This ability to discern serves to empower balance within the Law of Reciprocity, understanding healthy boundaries in both giving and receiving. It assures that the ability to be of service to the world is free from the energy of sacrifice of Self. Unblocking and activating this Energy Release Point monitors the flow of giving and receiving of nurturance and nourishment. It offers the opportunity to go within in order to reflect and study life. It allows for the connection to experience the loving, warm maternal embrace. It accesses an energy which is free from judgment and holds the seat of emotions and of Self in sacredness.

Disharmonies: *Self denial; abandonment; neediness; worry; lack of compassion; lack of empathy; judgmental attitudes towards self and/or others; restless sleep; separation anxiety; timidness.*

ST-17 Centre of the Breasts

Virtues: This Energy Release Point serves to clear dysfunctional emotional boundaries. It brings balance to the emotional life of the inner child who still tends to cling to a childlike dependent state. Centre of the Breasts brings the awareness that these dysfunctional emotional boundaries are in co-creation with the mother. In the early stages of life - in the womb, the life of the fetus depended upon nourishment for physical growth and vitality as fed through the umbilicus. The nourishment received through the mother, however, becomes more than just her nutritional intake.

Nourishment is also filtered through her thoughts and emotions in addition to the nutrients of the blood. This nourishment cannot help but feed the physical, emotional and mental needs of the developing baby. Once through the birth passage, the baby takes it's first breath and receives the spiritual inspiration and re-connection with the Divine Heavenly Essence. Spiritual nourishment then integrates with the Soul Essence and the Physical Body. The baby is then fed at the breast of the mother and learns how to navigate the boundaries of the physical plane of life through the healthy interaction and teachings of the mother. The baby hence learns nurturance to gentle weaning for a secure and healthy sense of Self - growing to a mature functioning adult. It is in accordance to the level of health or dysfunction, in regards to the appropriate sense of boundary and dependency at the breast, that will result in the level of healthy maturation or dysfunction of neediness in the later phases of life. Unblocking and activating this Energy Release Point brings awareness to behaviours resulting from inappropriate boundaries and insecurities. It empowers positive maturation and the acceptance of adult responsibilities in relation to the healing and integration of the unhealthy childhood identity.

Disharmonies: *Neediness; childlike behaviour and emotional manipulation; insecurity; inappropriate boundaries; co-dependency; possessiveness; control issues; isolation and solitary behaviour.*

ST-18 Root of the Breasts

Virtues: This Energy Release Point re-establishes the connection to maternal consciousness and brings one to reflection upon one's relationship to the feminine. In particular is the awareness of how one stands within the balance of giving and receiving. It is to connect with the root of source, the root which lays the foundation for one's ability to show nurturing care for others. The stomach is the source of nourishment and the Energy Release Channel of the stomach passes directly through the centre of the breast. As such, it speaks to the ability to connect with the maternal source of nourishment and the ability to draw on what is needed for vital energy to nourish oneself and others. Unblocking and activating this Energy Release

Point evokes the feeling of a time when one felt nurtured, safe and secure. From this feeling grows the confidence to reach deep into our roots to understand and know the core Self. From this depth of understanding we are empowered to grow into our abilities and reach out to the world. In this way, one can receive nourishment from the source within as well as nourishment from participation in life. It is from this wholeness of Being that one can truly produce and share the gifts necessary for the growth and benefit of others.

Disharmonies: *Feelings of childhood abandonment; alienation from mother or mothering roles; rejection of one's feminine aspects; feeling unloved; feeling unwanted; inability to ask for what one needs; internalized pain and trauma from childhood.*

ST- 19 Not At Ease

Virtues: This Energy Release Point expresses the ability to bring one to the state of being at ease. It releases worry and helps unwind tension held in the stomach and third energy centre which ultimately impacts the ability to digest. Not at Ease brings calmness to the mind, allowing for the acceptance of "it is as it is", from the point of view of trusting the Divine plan and perfect resolutions. Within the quality of acceptance one also develops the quality of forgiveness of Self and of others. Forgiveness is a powerful cleanser of the psyche, where thoughts are churned over obsessively. Unblocking and activating this Energy Release Point allows for a cleansing of the mind via the channel of forgiveness, ultimately resulting in calm and comfort. It is in this gentle space of serenity that one can surrender and accept the quality of ease and grace.

Disharmonies: *Overly dramatic engagement with life and taking things personally; worry and pensiveness; nervous stomach.*

ST-20 Receive and Support Fullness

Virtues: This Energy Release Point strengthens the ability to be generous from a place of inner abundance. When abundance is felt from within, the ability to see and appreciate the fullness of our surrounding environment and situation is strengthened. We are empowered to connect with the Creative Force, knowing that it is ever present and supportive. Feelings of satisfaction, pleasure, joy and wholeness resonate within the core of our Being and these same feelings are extended to others through our acts of generosity. Unblocking and activating this Energy Release Point connects us to the abundance of Source, that which is our Divine Right. It allows a flow of satisfaction from the completion of a job well done. It is to reap rewards from a harvest and to find contentment, security and stability. It harmonizes conflicts within our relationship towards giving and receiving so that we can come alive with the abundance and support of the Creative Force, restoring wholeness and completeness.

Disharmonies: *Wallowing in feelings of self pity; fear of lack; inability to give or share with others; emotionally needy; overeating as compensation for feeling empty inside; inability to feel nourished or nurtured; rejection of nourishment or nurturance from Self or others; feelings of not being enough; physical manifestations of anorexia, stomach pain, abdominal distention, poor appetite, rumbling intestines and difficult ingestion.*

ST-21 A Bridging Gateway

Virtues: This Energy Release Point brings harmony to opposites. It works with two Universal Laws: the Law of Polarity, allowing one to see from an elevated perspective both sides of a situation; and the Law of Rhythm, bringing regulation to the pendulum swing of movement between the two opposites. It is similar to standing in the middle of a bridge, observing and feeling the expanse and flow of motion. The Gateway on this bridge is the access to the flow of regulation similar to that of the function of a dam. When flow is reduced by the dam, there is calmness and tranquility. This provides the opportunity to view and digest life. When flow is augmented by the dam, there is motion and action to take the next steps. The gateway moves freely, adjusting to life circumstances so that one always feels centred, thus providing safe passage from one opposite to another. Unblocking and activating this Energy Release Point regulates the flow of movement. It allows for the constant fine tuning of energy streams setting the condition for perfect ebb and flow within a strong centre.

Disharmonies: *Stagnation on all levels - the physical digestive system as well as on the emotional, mental and spiritual planes; emotional blockages; extreme mood swings; being caught in turmoil; irritable bowel symptoms.*

ST-22 Illuminated Gate / Gate of Light

Virtues: This Energy Release Point is a gate of clarity and illumination bringing understanding to life experiences in order to transform these experiences into wisdom. This transformative process has the effect of bringing conscious awareness to one's thoughts, words and actions to an elevated perspective so that all the outward expressions of living are for the benefit of all. Illuminated Gate is a gateway which interconnects with the vast network of Energy Release Channels. This is much the same way that an individual interconnects with the web of humanity. The actions, thoughts and words of one have the ability to affect the whole. Therefore, the benefits of illumination and wisdom of one, affects and is felt by the ALL. Unblocking and activating this Energy Release Point empowers illumination and the manifestation of the highest potential. It brings awareness to darkness buried deep within, and through the alchemy of Light, transforms shadow into Light by the resolution of life lessons. Clarity is brought to a higher level of understanding of the Universal Law of Cause and Effect, of which both the Law of Karma and the Law of Accumulated Good are part. At this higher level of consciousness, realization of one's purpose and destiny manifests with clarity and potency.

Disharmonies: *Shutting the door on past experiences so as not to learn; inability to digest life manifesting in digestive issues such as diminishing* *appetite, constipation and diarrhea; inability to move through the stagnation of mundanity.*

ST- 23 Supreme Unity

Virtues: This Energy Release Point empowers the ability to integrate life experience in a way that promotes the strengthening and development of integrity. Within the energy of Supreme Unity, is the energy of the number one. The number one is represented as a vertical line connecting and bringing the energy of Heaven and the Creative Force down into the Earth via the physical vehicle of the Human. It is consciousness of the true Self, the I AM. It is essence and substance. It is primary existence. Supreme Unity brings this Divine consciousness into physicality to awaken the Self of the personality. This awakened Self awakens to unity consciousness and re-ignites within, the desire to strengthen integrity and re-alignment to the Soul's promptings. Unblocking and activating this Energy Release Point empowers the desire to return to one-ness, the ultimate unity of be-ing which is in alignment with Soul purpose. It facilitates the ability to follow through with our intentions to manifest our Divine potential. Integrity is strengthened and expressed outwardly as the alignment between our thoughts, our words, our heart and our actions integrate in unity and wholeness in the One.

Disharmonies: *Feeling burdened; feeling overwhelmed by life experiences; feeling scattered and without sense of direction; distracted by details; inability to see the whole picture; lack of integrity in thoughts, words and actions.*

ST-24 Lubricating Gateway

Virtues: This Energy Release Point activates the process of ingestion, digestion and assimilation. In this modern day of a technology driven society, there is a bombardment of the senses due to excess stimulation. This creates hypersensitivity as well as sensory congestion. Lubricating Gateway empowers the ability to slow down this active overload by harmonizing the organic living physical vehicle of the body within the context of a quick paced technology driven environment. The intention of lubrication is to provide smooth flow. This Energy Release Point assists one to slow down and find calm within the chaos. It creates the sense of ease, grace and simplicity. It allows for the ingestion of what is needed in terms of life experience as well as nutritional requirements for physical support. It provides the ability to flow with the pace of life and others. It empowers the ability to digest, retrieve and assimilate that which is beneficial and allows the non beneficial to move on with ease. Unblocking and activating this Energy Release Point honours the rhythmic flow of the individual and integrates it harmoniously with the pace of life. As the essential is assimilated, vitality, strength and stamina are also empowered. The overall sense of enriched nourishment flows through the whole body systems including the sensory systems. Lubrication Gateway allows one to move forward in ease and grace with the pace of life.

Disharmonies: *Heaviness; obstruction of thought processes; feeling revolted by the circumstances of life; inability to "stomach" life; feelings of being a "lost soul" due to over stimulation and sensory congestion; overwhelm due to excess stimulation; inability to focus and still the mind; unconscious patterns of eating such as: overeating, distracted eating, eating on the run, eating while stressed; psychic and physical indigestion.*

ST-25 Celestial Pivot

Virtues: This Energy Release Point empowers the quality of ease and grace through periods of growth and transition, by strengthening balance and centre as well as anchoring stability and grounding. A pivot is an axis upon which something turns. This Energy Release Point strengthens the connection between the Cosmic Pole Star and its direct relationship to the central axis of the Earth. It is an essential point, representing the grounded centre of the Earth around which all life revolves. Its location on the body is next to the navel, the centre of our being, on the border between two of the energetic cavities of the Three Elixir Fields. The mid cavity which assimilates nourishment and the lower cavity which eliminates the waste of that which no longer serves. It is said in ancient texts that the area above the Celestial Pivot is ruled by Celestial Energy; the area below the Celestial Pivot is ruled by Earthly Energy. The place where these energies intersect is the origin of Energy of men and women. It is the energy to move forward in present time, to create and to be a living expression. When one connects to this centre, one gracefully navigates life experience. Unblocking and activating this Energy Release Point harmonizes the ability to stay in rhythm and observe all angles and directions from a place of centre. It allows one to stay in balance within rhythmic swings between the poles of duality. It is an anchoring point from which we can pivot in a new direction in response to life experience. It allows for security as we continue to learn and grow.

Disharmonies: *Sensation that the Earth is moving from underneath one's feet; to postpone action; to procrastinate; to be caught in a cycle of inaction; to struggle; self doubt; to look back into the past with regret or uncertainty. Physical manifestation of rhythmic disorders such as found with Irritable Bowel Syndrome or inflammatory bowel disorders.*

ST- 26 Outer Mound to Understanding.

Virtues: This Energy Release Point brings one to the wisdom of what is ancient and sacred. In ancient times, people buried their ancestors in places known to be favourable for it's height, or as a place of victory from battle. A place of fortune and of good omen. These places were revered as sacred. It was further believed that when one stood on the mound of the ancestor, and connected with the wisdom found within the heart of the past generation, knowledge and understanding would illuminate within the heart of the seeker. From the top of the mound, the perspective and view of life has the ability to change in a way that answers both the formed and unformed question as to the understanding of life and one's place within it. Unblocking and activating this Energy Release

Point connects us to the heart of wisdom found within. It brings awareness and understanding to the Soul messages brought forth in dream time. It increases the perception of what is ancient and sacred. It strengthens the ability to learn from those who have passed, reflecting to us the power, strength and encouragement needed to fulfill destiny from those who have gone before.

Disharmonies: *Sense of separation; inability to connect to life purpose; boredom and apathy; disinterest in life and worldly affairs.*

ST-27 The Great Elder

Virtues: This Energy Release Point enhances the ability to find strength derived from wisdom gained by life experience. It is the ability to move through not only our personal experiences in a balanced way, but to also gain wisdom from the jewels passed on to us through our lineage. To gain wisdom from life experiences is in part derived from the ability to observe our patterns and our lifestyle habits as well as the patterns and lifestyle habits of our lineage or elders. Our innate constitutional physical vitality is derived from our genetics. From measurable observation, we can strengthen our weaknesses and balance ourselves by opening the gateway of our strengths to flow cyclically through the body and harmonize the whole. Unblocking and activating this Energy Release Point accesses the strength within, which supports and encourages our growth and evolution. It revitalizes through connection to our inner source of energy to give us stamina and balance.

Disharmonies: *Complete exhaustion; devitalization; habit of taking care of others without taking care of self; heroic tendencies as in helping in order to save others at the sacrifice of self; chronic fatigue; slow recovery after illness.*

ST-28 Water Path

Virtues: This Energy Release Point connects us to the flow of water and the purpose of water to nourish and sustain life. We are as water. We come from primordial source and as beings composed mostly of water, we are designed to flow upon our path. Following the way. The path of water can be likened to a channel, moving straight and true to the goal. At times, this channel can become blocked or broken. As a result, meandering detours are created as water continually seeks to arrive back to the Source. At other times, the water may dry up or flood over it's boundaries. Water is a live consciousness. Unblocking and activating this Energy Release Point helps one to understand the laws of Karma. It shows the playing out of Cause and Effect as a tool to bring awareness to our creation of life and the perceived obstacles that detour us from realizing our purpose. It brings awareness and healing to painful early emotions in regards to the parents with the realization that they are the teachers chosen to help us to learn and grow in our Soul evolution. It assists in balancing love forces of the heart and creating appropriate emotional boundaries.

Disharmonies: *Emptiness; dysfunctional outpouring of love; neediness; abandonment and lack of nurturance by the parents.*

ST-29 The Return

Virtues: This Energy Release Point speaks to the ability to return to, or to come back to something in order to flow forward. It is the ability to heal from inner reflection when re-evaluating and re-examining events of the past and having a wider perspective due to the wisdom of experience. This Energy Release Point also invokes the cyclic process of life, death and rebirth as a reflection of creation, transformation and receiving back. Giving becomes a process of the extension of creation. Consequently, receiving becomes the experience of the outcomes and benefits. This cycle nurtures the flow of wisdom and links the generations. The Elder expressing their advice and life perspectives to the younger members of family and community, who in turn continue the cycle for future generations. Unblocking and activating this Energy Release Point grants the space to pause and reflect. To turn around and look back in order to re-connect with our Soul Essence. From this perspective the impetus of growth is nourished from what has gone before in order to develop the opportunities which lie ahead. It is to return to the Source in order to renew life and living.

Disharmonies: *Inability to give and to receive; inability to create; inability to move forward towards change; disrupted cycles such as sleep or menstrual; inability to reflect and observe life in order to learn and grow.*

ST-30 Rushing Energy / Thoroughfare of Energy

Virtues: This Energy Release Point has the ability to harmonize energy that has a tendency to rise up with sudden swiftness. It is a modulator or balancer which calms the rush and allows for a smooth flow of energy that brings nourishment to the heart and calmness to the mind. Within this process, this Energy Release Point clears the pathway from the heart to the mind, allowing free flow through the neck, where panic energy can gather and re-route it to where it belongs - in the third energy centre. The empowerment of the third energy centre allows for clearly directed will forces. By conscious connection to the will, one can then restore their authentic power, a power which releases control, manipulation or passivity when in relationship with others. Unblocking and activating this Energy Release Point harmonizes energy to empower life. It calms the emotional body and balances any feeling that produces agitation. It promotes self care which integrates nurturance, as well as nourishment received from positive life experiences. It helps one to trust in the smooth unfolding of life's path. It assists in the ability to open emotionally and form deep committed intimate relationships, as well as facilitates the integration of spiritual life forces within the physical being.

Disharmonies: *Overwhelm; fear; fear of exposure; vulnerability; intimacy issues; panic; anxiety; suppressed sexuality; feelings of isolation and separation; digestive disorders leading to acid reflux; heart palpitations; hot flashes; gynaecological disorders; lower abdominal pain; impotence; hunger with no desire to eat.*

ST-31 Network of Strength / Thigh Gate

Virtues: This Energy Release Point assists in the support of the physical body, giving it strength and flexibility. It is similar to a gateway opening to a great vital energy that allows us to leap out into the world and take it on. The virtue of flexibility allows us to navigate through obstacles and bends in the road. The virtue of strength supports perseverance in fulfilling our goals and manifesting vision. Unblocking and activating this Energy Release Point helps put our ideas and visions into action, so that we can spring forth and embrace life with flexibility and joy.

Disharmonies: *Iron willed; inflexible; inability to accept help from others resulting in exhaustion; martyrdom and self sacrificial behaviour. Physical manifestation of blocked circulation in the legs; leg pain; restricted hip movement and cold in the knees.*

ST-32 Crouching Hare

Virtues: This Energy Release Point is located in the centre of the thigh muscle. The shape of the muscle at this point resembles that of a crouching hare. The visualization of this image brings forward the qualities of the hare, such as it's agility and speed. A hare has great sensitivity, it can sense what is coming and as such, knows how to hide in order to save itself. The hare does not sacrifice itself. The hare is a complex animal that has many symbols. In Ancient Greece, it was the symbol of the goddess Hecate who lived in the underworld where she oversaw the rituals of purification as well as magical invocations. From this, we view the hare as a symbol of magical luck as well as purification and rebirth. Indeed, the hare has the remarkable ability to reproduce, thereby bringing the association of fertility and creativity. In Ancient Egypt, the hare is depicted in hieroglyphs associated with the concept of Being. In Ancient China, the hare is one of the twelve astrological signs and considered to be a most fortunate sign. Those born in the sign of the Hare had the ability to possess the powers of the moon. The hare brings the qualities of sensitivity, intuition, artistry and ambition. In Europe, the hare is magical in that it's coat could change colour with the changing of the seasons. In addition, it was usually seen in the early mornings or at twilight and thus, had the ability to move between the physical world and the Fairy kingdom. Unblocking and activating this Energy Release Point helps one to understand the limits of physicality as well as to have a healthy recognition of one's own needs. It brings to full awareness the qualities of one's gifts of creativity so that the connection to purpose is empowered. It is this connection to our creative authentic Being that serves to strengthen the limbs to carry out the directives of the Soul plan. It brings forward a rebirthing energy. It facilitates the ability to manifest decisive action towards our goals with ease, respecting the physical body and without sacrifice to our vitality and integrity.

Disharmonies: *Exhaustion; over exertion; workaholic syndrome; excessive worry; catering to the needs of others; neediness; blocked creativity; inflexibility; lack of strength or energy to manifest vision; lack of sensitivity; blocked intuition.*

ST-33 Market of the Mysterious Feminine

Virtues: This Energy Release Point brings to understanding the sacredness of ritual and ceremony. It assists in being open to receive the gifts from the heavenly realms and to integrate them within. Through alchemy, vitality draws forth sacred action for manifested creation. It is important to honour this process of creation, to have ceremony in recognition of its realization. Ceremony acknowledges the virtue of self worth and reinforces sacredness. Unblocking and activating this Energy Release Point brings the acceptance of one's unique individuality, builds self-worth and assists in connecting to inner divinity. From this place of truth, one is empowered to produce and to share one's gifts with others.

Disharmonies: *Unworthiness; distorted sense of Self; self-effacement; inability to express and share one's gifts.*

ST-34 Beam Mound

Virtues: This Energy Release Point helps bring strength, energy and enthusiasm to be involved in the day to day living of life. It allows one to move into centre, where, through tranquility and calmness, one develops mindfulness. In the state of mindfulness, perception becomes finely tuned.

It becomes easier to slow down the input of life. It allows for discernment and enhances the ability to take in what is beneficial for nurturance and nourishment. A beautiful circle of restoration of vitality and joyful enthusiasm is created: move into centre, find tranquility and calm, develop mindfulness, fine tune perception, recognize joy in the task, move back into centre and continue the cycle. Beam Mound empowers the ability to transform the mundane and perceived burdens in order to move more freely in life. Unblocking and activating this Energy Release Point assists in releasing the feeling of being encumbered. It helps one to rise above mundanity to see the bigger picture in life, from a clear vantage point of the elevated perspective of the mound. In this way one can perceive the path that leads to the manifestation of goals. As the Essential Self rediscovers its innate vitality through joyful living, the ability to nurture oneself and others evolves in a balanced way.

Disharmonies: *Bitterness and resentment; fatigue and weariness; excessive consumption in an attempt to feel satisfied; dysfunctional relationship to food; over-eating; eating too quickly.*

ST-35 Calf's Nose

Virtues: This Energy Release Point restores the feelings of support and love, such as the experience of a child within a healthy functioning family. Through a healthy maturation process of embracing both the feminine and masculine aspects of Self, the child grows into a fully functioning adult who is able to face responsibilities as a citizen of the world. This is similar to the healthy maturation of a calf. The growth into the male bull has the qualities of bringing nourishment through slaughter - that is, bringing fertility and gifts through sacrifice. The growth into the female cow brings the qualities of nourishment through non-violence and nurturance. By integrating these two opposites, one learns to distinguish service from servitude and sympathy from compassion. By learning to discern in this way, the ability to trust in the process of life experience becomes joyful and the facility to release perceived burdens becomes easy. Unblocking and activating this Energy Release Point builds inner fortitude and perseverance to continue carrying both physical and emotional loads with the attitude of enthusiasm. It helps one to face responsibilities by restoring childlike wonder, awe and joy within a healthy functioning adult.

Disharmonies: *Sore tired body; achy knees; lack of enthusiasm for doing and serving; sacrificial behaviour; subservience; mistrust of the motives of others; fear; cynicism to life.*

ST-36 Leg Three Miles / Lower Tomb / Ghost Evil

Virtues: This Energy Release Point nourishes the muscles and strengthens the ability to feel grounded, centred and stable. When one is grounded and centred, the ability to align one's thoughts, intentions and actions evolves with more clarity and facility. This alignment is an essential component in bringing forward the manifestation of action, gifts and talents. Also being grounded and centred endows us with the strength and ability to share these gifts and talents with the world community for the betterment of humanity. Unblocking and activating this Energy Release Point facilitates connection to the centred Being. It serves to fully integrate the Spiritual Self with the Physical Self in order to flow with direct and purposeful action of Destiny. It strengthens the awareness and realization that there are gifts that only you can bring to the world. That you are an essential part of the plan within the interconnected web of humanity, earth, animal, mineral and plant kingdom. This powerful Release Point enables the body to physically continue despite all obstacles and hindrances. As this Point's alternative name Lower Tomb implies, it is understood that sometimes in order to discover one's purpose one may need to go deep within. The journey inwards has the ability to draw out and heal painful darkness that the psyche has stuffed down in the shadows. However it is through this journey of pain that one can discover the buried jewels and treasure. Unblocking and activating this Energy Release Point, in this context, strengthens the ability to draw on the wealth of family lineage and the wisdom of genetic history in order to resurrect the treasure. The name, Ghost Evil, is to discern the distractions which seduce you from the fulfillment of your life's purpose. Unblocking and activating this Energy Release

Point with this intention is to strengthen the ability to stay focused and on course.

Disharmonies: *Over-consumption; materialistic view; inflexible; being stuck; apathy and lacking of motivation; depletion; stubborn; lethargic; unwilling or unable to move from current circumstances; compromise of position in order to please others; ingratiating behaviour which undermines one's integrity leading to physical depletion; overcome by shadow aspects; muscle weakness; pain in the knees.*

ST-37 Upper Great Void / Upper Purity

Virtues: This Energy Release Point addresses the quality of non-attachment and contentment. The Upper Great Void is the expression of the God-force. It is indescribable and unknowable. It is the space of Oneness with the source of ALL THAT IS. It represents the Cosmic Egg from where all things come. It denotes absolute freedom from every limitation. It is infinite and eternal Conscious Energy which, in itself, is No-Thing manifested in everything. Boundless, infinite potential - the base of all consciousness. Unblocking and activating this Energy Release Point strengthens the ability to connect to this God-force energy via inspiration. It brings a sense of security and trust that one is always supported and connected to the spiritual world where there is eternal freedom in the expression of Light. It brings contentment, stability and strength to move through painful experiences in order to heal and release these attachments to the pain of one's personal story.

Disharmonies: *Holding on to that which has lost its value as a habitual way of avoiding the pain of loss; deep seated grief; difficulty in sorting and letting go in life; physical manifestations of digestive issues and fluctuating constipation and diarrhea.*

ST-38 Lines Opening

Virtues: This Energy Release Point allows for the lines and branches to higher thought process to open so that clarity and focus can prevail. Such clarity sets into motion the flow of what is extraneous to release and frees the mind to find calm and tranquility. In the state of calm and tranquility, one can access higher thought. Lines Opening empowers the strength of integration of the higher mental bodies with the physical system so that ideas and speech co-ordinate in a coherent manner. Unblocking and activating this Energy Release Point enhances communication through the building of courage and strengthening of stability. This enhancement allows for Spirit to radiate through the personality for inspired and continual growth.

Disharmonies: *Overthinking; inability to organize clear, cohesive thought; inability to take action; disorganized communication; mental confusion; overwhelm; physical, mental and emotional toxicity manifesting into problems with elimination: boils, skin lesions for example; feelings of disgust; feelings of bitterness; feelings of disdain.*

ST- 39 Lower Great Void

Virtues: This Energy Release Point creates the stream of energy connecting the Upper Great Void into the Lower Great Void. It is movement from the macrocosm of the Universal All into the microcosm of the incarnated Spiritual Being. This connection reinforces the remembrance of the One, of being in Unity with ALL That Is. Unblocking and activating this Energy Release Point assists one to feel protected and guided, safe and secure. It is when one can sit in this space and meditate on the Void of existential emptiness that we can tap into the vitality of the Creative Force and channel it in a positive way for the benefit of humanity. It strengthens the connection to a higher aspect of Self, bringing, as result, mental clarity of purpose and joy in the process of Soul evolution.

Disharmonies: *Anxiety; mania; no pleasure in eating; lack of clarity seen as mixed messages; joylessness; vulnerability.*

ST-40 Abundant Splendour

Virtues: This Energy Release Point strengthens our connection to reveal and acknowledge our intrinsic self worth. When self worth is acknowledged, we are impelled to look into our authentic selves and acknowledge our qualities and gifts. Inspiring us to seek further and align with our purpose as directed by Soul vision. Glimpsing into the authentic self unlocks the reality of our potential. It allows one to sense and see a vision of the future - a vision of life which is free from struggle and hardship. It is this vision which motivates. It allows the balance between calmness and gathering potential and vision with the manifestation of action through creative drive. It is a vision of joy, abundance and prosperity. It is the ability to taste of the fruits of ones labour and be filled with satisfaction and contentment. Unblocking and activating this Energy Release Point stimulates and brings access to a source of energy. An energy which empowers contentment, vitality, abundance and prosperity from the alignment of heavenly purpose manifested by physical action in the material world.

Disharmonies: *Excessive weight; insatiable appetite; selfishness; neediness; ingratiation; unworthiness, overwhelm; feeling burdened by friends, family, and/or career; loss of momentum and motivation to create and flow with life; inability to connect with the sense of satisfaction upon the completion of a project.*

ST-41 Stream of Release

Virtues: This Energy Release Point processes the pain of past experiences and strengthens fiery energy to break through burdens and stagnation. By consequence this fired up energy creates a release. This release can sometimes show as a torrent of tears. Stream of Release re-establishes the momentum and flow of the assimilation of inspiration and of life; the integration of nourishment in order to flow new creation and manifestation;

as well as the elimination of the non-beneficial and the extraneous which do not serve the Divine Plan for our life. The self imposed constraints to forward motion and manifestation of desires are unfastened and removed. The ability to understand and solve our perceived problems is enhanced as the virtues of clarity, understanding, compassion and co-operation are restored. Unblocking and activating this Energy Release Point allows for the untying of constraints for beneficial release. A release which heals and restores flow to active and conscious participation in our co-creation with the Divine for manifestation of living joy. Stream of Release creates connection to the world leading to renewed interest and enthusiasm for life. The restoration of contentment as well as enthusiasm for joyful service balanced with the principles of giving and receiving.

Disharmonies: *Inability to let go of pain; inability to learn from the past and move forward; inability to digest and receive nourishment from life manifesting in digestive disorders; unexplained weight gain or weight loss; lack of interest in life and others; discontent; dissatisfaction; hunger after eating; manic behaviour showing as extreme self centre; obsessions regarding one's own needs and verbal diarrhea.*

ST-42 Meet and Surrender

Virtues: This Energy Release Point allows one to find balanced strength. It is to connect with clarity to the knowledge of when to surrender. The act of surrendering is an act of strength. It takes strength and courage for the personality to release negative ego, for negative ego wishes to battle through on its continual impulse to seek, dominate and control. Through Meet and Surrender, the personality finds connection with the Higher Self and is impelled to shift forward in its evolution towards wholeness. It releases the need to exert will forces on Self and on others. Unblocking and activating this Energy Release Point assists one to find equanimity with Self and others. It provides the courage to shift and make changes directed from within. It brings forward realizations that true freedom is found when conditions to living are released and barriers to the Higher Self are dissolved through the qualities of grace and forgiveness. Meet and

Surrender brings forward the positive attributes of surrender. It provides balance, stability and centre as one flows into wholeness and completion.

Disharmonies: *Over-striving without mindfulness to the needs of the body; forcing one's will onto others; desire to be in control and dominate; intolerant to the individuality of others.*

ST-43 Sinking Valley

Virtues: This Energy Release Point strengthens the ability to digest and assimilate life by empowering integrity and alignment to purpose. It is often observed that as one compromises in integrity or detours from alignment, their world begins to crumble and fall apart. Life becomes struggle and challenges seem insurmountable and unavoidable. The name Sinking Valley evokes the image of a crumbling foundation, the erosion of banks and barriers leading to the ultimate collapse of integrity. Unblocking and activating this Energy Release Point assists one to stay in integrity and to hold one's centre. The ability to hold centre is, by direct connection and alignment, to the central pillar of strength - the strength of which is derived precisely by the alignment of one's little will to the Divine Will. It brings realization that a body is strong, healthy and vital only by the honouring of one's innate sense of purpose. It is then recognizing that this innate sense of purpose is always in balance with one's authentic truth. This balance promotes self care and nurturance as essential qualities to the continuation of this balance. Self care and nurturance become priorities in life so that the path becomes clear. These qualities serve to promote uprightness and self assertion as we strive towards our goals in a centred and grounded way, being the example and way- shower to others.

Disharmonies: *Easily distracted from goals leading to apathy and depression; difficulty staying on task; feelings of overwhelm; sinking in despair; loss of expression of purpose; loss of sense of purpose; inability to process life; Physical symptoms of prolapses of the lower body organs.*

ST-44 Inner Courtyard

Virtues: This Energy Release Point prepares and quiets the mind for meditation by going inwards and connecting with a courtyard of calm. Within this courtyard there is a fountain of water. The movement of water allows for the flow of spirit to refresh and regenerate our whole body systems within a place of beauty. It empowers the quality of reflection by calming overactive thoughts. Inner Courtyard brings about a state of incubation, a time of rest before the seeding of high creative potential. It is a time of allowing the integration of all the previous accomplishments to take effect and to give time for the fruits of labour to nourish us with their wholeness. Unblocking and activating this Energy Release Point brings about a deep meditative state so that the divine seeds of inspiration can incubate in preparation for transformative states of growth.

Disharmonies: *Greed and lust for possessions and power; materialism and congestion; being overcome with personal needs and desires; inability to transform and release negative ego; worry; obsession; failure to embrace spirit; nightmares.*

ST- 45 Hard Bargain

Virtues: This Energy Release Point assists in developing flexibility within the quality of reciprocity. It establishes a functional balance in our ability to give and our ability to receive. Often times, the ability to reciprocate is based upon the ability of the Self to accept oneself with all of one's imperfections. In this case, it is important to release harsh judgmental attitudes towards Self and learn forgiveness. Through forgiveness, one can more easily accept nourishment from Self and subsequently open up to accept and receive nourishment from others. Once this is established, the ability to reciprocate in turn is facilitated. One then finds within a flexibility to life, a flow, an ease and grace. Unblocking and activating this Energy Release Point allows for the flow of nourishment from the essentials derived from life experience. It empowers the ability to receive that which is substantial. This activation encompasses the ability to seize the jewels of life experiences in order to realize our potential and to eliminate the non-essential and non-beneficial. In this way we can build on the elements that serve and enrich us in order to be of service to others. As one builds generosity and reciprocity, one creates and strengthens the resonant light frequencies within so that buoyancy and lightness in the heart is the natural condition of living.

Disharmonies: *Tendency towards harsh judgment of Self and others; inability to forgive; over consumption of goods; overly materialistic clinging to wealth and possessions; dissatisfaction; addictions to alcohol, seen as a form of drowning our sorrows or addiction to shopping, seen as a way to fill insatiable needs; victim mentality.*

Portraits of the Energy Release
Points for the Energy Release
Channel of the Spleen

SP- 1 Hidden White / Ghost Eye

Virtues: This Energy Release Point empowers the feeling of freedom to open up to receive nourishment from life. It supplies the strength needed to find and stay in centre and integrity. It is located on the foot, and as such, is the intermediary between the vision of Soul expression made physical and the stepping into the vision of purpose. It creates balance between the physical plane of existence, where one must do the mundane to live the earthly life, and the plane of celestial harmony, where one recognizes a state of being that is filled with love, joy and ease. When one connects with Hidden White, one also connects to the symbol of purity. The purity that comes when viewing oneself as sacred. Embracing sacredness allows the freedom to become who we are so that life becomes a joyful expression of purpose. Unblocking and activating this Energy Release Point opens us up to new ideas and direction, motivating us to put our Soul visions into actions. It serves to balance strength, flexibility and emotional stability. It assists to recognize and stand up to our own needs in keeping with clarity of thought and vision. The alternate name, Ghost Eye, is in reference to this Energy Release Point being a ghost point on the body. A place on the body where an entity enters and seemingly drains one of all vitality. Unblocking and activating with the intention of Ghost Eye is to address the disfunction of feeling extraordinarily drained for unknown reasons as well as solving mysterious disorders of the blood leading to weakness.

Disharmonies: *Lack of assertiveness; ingratiating behaviour towards others to avoid anger and conflict; disorganization; inability to feel grounded or centred; slow thought processes; lethargy; boredom; difficulty in concentration; mental fogginess; obsessive thoughts; dreamy disposition and vivid fantasy life; restless mind; insomnia; blood disorders such as trouble with blood coagulation, inability to stop bleeding; muscle and sinew weakness; weakness of the internal organs; acid reflux; heartburn; bitter and sour taste in the mouth.*

SP-2 Great Metropolis

Virtues: This Energy Release Point embodies the concept of community life where there are exchanges and heartfelt sharing with people. It brings forward the awareness of the preciousness of humanity and strengthens the desire to participate in life. Within community there is a busy-ness of gatherings and exchanges for mutual benefits. Through the balanced flow of giving and receiving, vitality is constantly being spent and regenerated. This balanced exchange brings a wholeness and solidity. Life flows and one receives nourishment through loving connection with friends, family and creative pursuits. Fulfillment, contentment and joy abound as one opens wholeheartedly and extends love to humanity while receiving the inflow of the gifts of exchange. Unblocking and activating this Energy Release Point opens our hearts to warmth and positive exchanges within our relationships. It allows us to be the best of ourselves through the care of ourselves. It is to see the beauty and good in all things and circumstances of life so that our hearts fill with compassionate understanding and love.

Disharmonies: *Feelings of burden; feelings of obligation towards friends and family; inability to make clear decisions; over extending ourselves leading to self sacrifice and martyrdom; feeling listless and sluggish; passivity; social alienation; depletion; lack of fulfillment; having a hungry heart; discontent. Physical manifestation of fibromyalgia; burning pain in the muscles; excessive weight gain.*

SP-3 Supreme White / Venus

Virtues: This Energy Release Point addresses the condition of the lifestream in embodiment. It is to be fully grounded with the spirit fully in the body so that actions taken and visions manifested come from a centre of self love, self respect, self honour, self nourishment and nurturance, purity and humility. These conditions are of the highest impeccability, integrity and discernment. In this way, one can love, respect, honour, nourish and nurture humanity and the Earth. This Energy Release Point is located on the foot. Unblocking and activating Supreme White brings a surge of vitality and allows for the firm planting of steady feet walking the path, fulfilling purpose and destiny through connection to one's true Essence.

Disharmonies: *Feeling burdened; being needy; ungrateful; low self-esteem; lack of self love; doormat syndrome; lack of integrity and core values; poor relationship with mother; constant caretaker with depletion due to lack of self care; inability to receive; martyrdom.*

SP- 4 Yellow Emperor / Grandparent-Grandchild

Virtues: This Energy Release Point is the only Energy Release Point on the body with a royal name. It speaks to human history that is found in mythology. In this mythology one finds a distant Divine ancestor representing Heaven, as well as a distant ancestor representing Earth. In this respect it serves to unify the light of the Mind of Heaven with the passion of the Heart of Earth. It is to be unselfish, to be open to all and to create and share posterity for the benefit of humanity. This Energy Release Point also is the family name of the mythological Yellow Emperor who ruled China for 100 years from 2697 BC to 2597 BC. It is symbolic of gold, royalty, merit, youth, virginity, happiness and fertility. It is the Yellow Emperor that received ancient wisdom of medicine to help ease the suffering of his people. He taught them to be stewards of the Earth and the Earth in turn would nourish the nation. By tending the Earth and teaching future generations the ability to do the same, the Emperor could be assured that prosperity, stability and abundance would be the birthright of all the descendants of his people. In this way, future generations would continually reap the riches of the harvests and as such this would be the inheritance of the royal treasury. Unblocking and activating this Energy Release Point empowers the unification of generations. It forms a bridge between the wisdom of the past and brings hope for the future. It unites and strengthens the ability to act in accordance to the heart's passion while strengthening the forces of will. Yellow Emperor combines strength with wisdom and creates hope and optimism for the future generations in order for humanity to continue the journey.

Disharmonies: *Dysfunctional comfort seeking behaviour; addictions or addictive behaviour; being disheartened and depressed; hopelessness; pessimism and despair; conflict with images of authority; alienation from the past; disconnection with genetic lineage; unconscious wasteful behaviour in regards to environmental issues; disconnection from nature; unconscious exploitative behaviours in regards to nature.*

SP-5 Merchant Mound

Virtues: This Energy Release Point is both cleansing and calming and assists in re-energizing the digestive process. The musical note associated with this point is in resonance with that of the element metal and the alchemical process, the sound which brings the virtues of strength, clarity, harmony and righteousness. The ability to discern truths from untruths; to weigh choices and eliminate non-essentials is heightened. Each Energy Release Channel speaks to a fundamental element of alchemy. This Energy Release Channel of the Spleen speaks to the Earth Element - the centre and point of stillness within the energy of movement. All things move, however there is a calm centre, a place of non-movement; an eternal stillness or existential emptiness where alchemy manifests. These points show up in specific times, such as periods of transition like equinox and solstices, midnight and noon. This Energy Release Point speaks of this centre of calm, the point just before the return, creating a space where discussion, deliberation, clarity are examined and ideas and knowledge are exchanged. A space/time such as that in the time of the Ancients: Pythagorus or Confucius. A place of wisdom teachers. This Energy Release Point empowers harmony, balance and retainment of what is valuable and releases the extraneous.

Disharmonies: *Feelings of being stuck in life; poor self image; feelings of worthlessness; overeating; binging; lethargy. Physically these imbalances can present as digestive disorders; diarrhea embodying grief and weeping (from the lower orifice); constipation embodying congestion; excessive weight.*

SP-6 Union of the Three Feminine Mysteries

Virtues: This Energy Release Point enhances three Divine Mysteries: the storage and distribution of Spirit; the connection with Spirit; the Flowing with Spirit. When these three mysteries are brought together for unification and integration, they amplify strength and vibrancy. The number three is symbolic for understanding the components necessary for brilliant creativity. It conveys the idea that through growth found in creative expression, comes perfect manifestation as inspired by the movement of Spirit. Unblocking and activating this Energy Release Point enhances the action of the Three Treasures, that of receiving inspiration of Heaven and mingling it with vitality drawn of the Earth so that passionate energy, fuelled by the Heart of Desire, can evolve and move into full expression of the manifestation of potential.

Disharmonies: *Deep depression; desperation; wanting to run away from a situation, circumstance, people, place or thing; frustration to the point of rebelliousness.*

SP- 7 Leaking Valley

Virtues: This Energy Release Point evokes the image of a lush valley that is oozing with richness of material. This nutrient rich material is to be transported out of the valley to nourish areas that are otherwise impoverished in order to bring life, growth and nourishment to the populace. This image is a metaphor for the altruistic impulse found within when waiting is over. The talents and gifts that we wish to offer are developed and ready to move out and expand to joyful service. Ignoring the impulse to serve and distribute one's gifts becomes draining and as a consequence, the energy of stagnation and sluggishness ensue. Over time, the ability to receive and process information and nutrients becomes blocked and the whole body systems slow down in response. Unblocking and activating this Energy Release Point fuels the movement necessary to share ourselves with others. It sparks the altruistic impulses to be involved with the world, develop compassion and serve joyfully. It harmonizes the balance between storing and sitting on our potential, with sharing ourselves outwardly, in active transformation of potential into manifestation of reality.

Disharmonies: *Easily depleted or exhausted; chronic fatigue; excessive need to give or receive sympathy; craving sugar to ease the need to satisfy something more; neediness; nostalgia and sentimentality; imbalances in the immune system; leaky gut syndrome.*

SP-8 Earth Motivator

Virtues: This Energy Release Point has a dual function in that it can stimulate motivation and willingness to participate in life or it can help the constant do-er to relax. Earth Motivator brings the opportunity to seize the day and spring into joyous action. It brings consciousness to activity so that there is mindfulness and awareness to boundaries of either overdoing or constant doing. Life is about breathing in experiences as well as processing and integrating them into consciousness. It is important to honour the physical needs of the body through proper rest and nutrition as well as play and creative connection. Through conscious awareness, the ability to adapt to circumstances as they present is enhanced. It becomes a knowing of when to extend ourselves and nurture others and when to receive nourishment in return. It means being attentive to the needs of others as well as ourselves. Unblocking and activating this Energy Release Point brings energy to move through lethargy and depletion so that vitality and enthusiasm can be restored. It serves to balance overactive tendencies that eventually lead to burnout and exhaustion, by allowing one to consciously let go of old habits and lifestyles that deplete life forces. It brings about the inner realization on how to approach life in a way that nourishes the Soul.

Disharmonies: *Polarization of energy such as having inertia or the inability to slow down; feeling heavy, lethargic and bored; feeling bogged down and overwhelmed because of constant doing.*

SP-9 Feminine Spring Mound

Virtues: This Energy Release Point has the ability to bring vitality and its energetic flow to every part of the body, in particular to the internal organs. It is strengthening vitality, it is life giving and life renewing. It revitalizes and refreshes in the same way that a spring bursts through the earth in vibrant, sparkling clarity. Connecting to this spring allows for the continual flow of vital energy. Energy that is needed to move forward with the strength to break through obstacles that may come our way. It nourishes life experiences so that they may thrive in richness and continue to enhance vitality in return. Unblocking and activating this Energy Release Point accesses our inner Source. A Source that is renewed by the Source of the ALL That Is. It brings forward the mysteries of the Fountain of Youth - the Elixir of vitality and regeneration. Tapping into this Source gives strength and flow to follow one's path in service, back to Source.

Disharmonies: *Disappointment; lack of compassion; inability to open and receive the blessings that surround us; hardened attitude towards the world; unfulfilled desires leading to discontent and dissatisfaction; lethargy; boredom; fear of life; obsessive worry; dysfunctional relationship between caring for self and caring for others. Physical manifestation for women: uterine fibroids and gynaecological disorders.*

SP-10 Sea of Blood / Hundred Insect Nest

Virtues: This Energy Release Point strengthens the energy needed to circulate vital sources of nourishment that is found and transported in the blood. By stimulating this energy, the ability to connect and flow creativity and develop physical vigour and strength is enhanced. Fertility in all aspects - thought and creative processes as well as reproduction and instinct is applied, in order to channel and produce the desired effects. Unblocking and activating this Energy Release Point serves to physically revitalize the life giving circulatory forces of the blood. It also assists in calming agitation in the blood, which mirrors agitation of the mind, as well as physical itchiness of the skin. By consequence, the feelings of nurturance, love and support are strengthened. It facilitates the ability to receive and use nourishment for the benefit of creation. It helps one to explore within to find the source of disharmony which dulled the circulation of life giving vitality in the first place.

Disharmonies: *Eating disorders; chronic malnutrition; imbalanced vegetarian and vegan practices; scarcity and lack; survival consciousness; poverty consciousness; complete exhaustion after a long struggle or illness; great depletion from substantial blood loss; blood based gynaecological disorders such as excessive uterine bleeding; skin lesions and intolerable itchiness.*

SP-11 Winnower Basket Gate

Virtues: This Energy Release Point evokes the image of a winnower carrying his bamboo basket to the gateway of a marketplace. The Winnower's Basket is extraordinary. It is made of strong bamboo, therefore it can hold an abundant harvest. The fact that it serves to separate the chaff and debris from the grain shows the function of separating the essential from the inessential. The winnower transports this basket full of the fruits of labour to the market for the benefit of the greater community, knowing that the exchange will honour the labour and dedication to his/her role. Unblocking and activating this Energy Release Point brings the gifts of one's dedication to purpose through the gateway so that one can access great stores of vitality and nourishment for the body. The gateway is such that it regulates not only the proper amount of energy needed to revitalize the body, but also where the energy needs to go in order to keep the physical body in a harmonious state. Winnower Basket Gate accesses the strength of a bamboo basket. A basket which is filled with resources which serve to bring stability and vitality, so that in turn we can better serve humanity.

Disharmonies: *Depletion and exhaustion; martyrdom; servitude; inability to fully recuperate; physical manifestations include difficult urination; painful swelling in the groin area; impairment and pain in the lower limbs.*

SP-12 Rushing Gate / Palace of Motherly Compassion / Palace of Charity

Virtues: This Energy Release Point allows for the integration of the two opposite ends of the poles: that of Heaven and that of Earth. The pole is an axis, with Heaven and Earth on two opposite sides with a swirling vortex of energy keeping them apart. At the same time, this swirling vortex of energy is penetrated by Heaven and Earth. To access this energy is similar to opening a gate. This gate is a portal to a whirling surge of energy which fuels and empowers the body to forge ahead and carry on its mission. This mission is often associated with one's service to humanity. As Palace of Motherly Compassion, one draws on the wisdom of Ancients and shaman tradition of Earth Mother. In this tradition, there is harmony and balance within the mother/child relationship. This Earth Mother is bountiful, providing the needs for all her children. She is the symbol of protection, fertility and sustenance. The Earth Mother as the Divine Mother embodies compassion and mercy. The Divine Mother as world mother expresses the virtues of charity and altruism, hence the third name for this Energy Release Point, Palace of Charity. The virtue of charity is said to be the mother of all virtues and is often exemplified through the acts of kindness and of giving to those whose needs are more dire than one's own. Charity exemplifies the Love of the Creative Force, representing a bond between the God-force and humankind. Unblocking and Activating this Energy Release Point accesses the vital energy needed to carry out the directives of the Higher Self as it pertains to living altruistic service, while at the same time engendering the ability to protect one's vitality from overuse and depletion. It further allows one to care for others, trusting in the most benevolent outcome for continual support from the Divine.

Disharmonies: *Depletion of vitality when in service to others; actions and generosity motivated from personal agenda; dysfunctional nurturing tendencies based on worry; absorbing worry and negativity from mother while in utero; obsessive compulsive disorders; conditional love; distortions in survival consciousness leading to the inability to give or do service to others; fear of lack; poverty consciousness.*

SP-13 Official Residence, Our Home

Virtues: This Energy Release Point allows for transformation. A healthy and easy transformation which comes from being connected to a stabilized strength of home in the centre of our Being. It promotes harmony and calm allowing for the energy of being present. When one is fully present, one can solidify a vision of creativity and manifest a purpose filled life. Unblocking and activating this Energy Release Point allows one to connect to this place of wellbeing, empowering refinement of the quality of care and nurturance one gives to oneself, as well as strengthening the physical condition of the body.

Disharmonies: *Scattered thinking and an overactive mind; feeling lost like a child and looking for help. Physically this Energy Release Point helps with abdominal fullness and distention, abdominal pain and constipation.*

SP-14 Abdomen Knot

Virtues: This Energy Release Point empowers our connection to the time in the womb. The time before earthly life, a place where one can feel safe and secure. The quality of being able to feel safe, secure, nourished, supported and loved is measured in relation to this womb experience. Should this womb time be a place of pain and stress, we can re-connect and understand core experiences that define our emotional history in relationship to that of our parents. From this understanding one can see a bigger picture, reclaim the past and move towards compassionate awareness of our humanity. This empowers the realization that we have chosen our experiences in order to learn, grow and experience a broad range of human emotions. Unblocking and activating this Energy Release Point serves to untie knots that block the expression of painful emotions in order to allow healing of the pain and reconnection to the optimum. The optimum being a time of spiritual and physical nurturance that is untainted by life's painful experiences. Ultimately, this brings a sense of physical nurturance and belonging. The ability to commit to a community, find family and feel a sense of one's place becomes more feasible. It promotes a steady centre and sense of safety so that one may more fully embrace life.

Disharmonies: *Repression of powerful emotions; inability to forgive others; dysfunctional relationship to both the feminine aspects and masculine aspects of Self; disempowerment and victim mentality; blame; hostile projections; feelings of mistrust.*

SP-15 Great Horizontal

Virtues: This Energy Release Point promotes the firmness of support derived from standing on a strong foundation. This foundation is built on life experiences. When one goes through life feeling the support of the masculine in particular, there is an energy of strength and unwavering trust that all will proceed with positive intention for benevolence and joy. Likewise, when this is integrated with the support of the feminine Earth, we are empowered to stand firmly knowing that we are provided for and protected. This ensures healthy self sufficiency. When one integrates both these feminine and masculine aspects, one is rewarded with a renewed sense of vitality. The ability to form healthy boundaries when in service to others and receive the exchange flows naturally and with ease. It can also be said that life experiences can be obscured by the energy of pain. Pain, such as sadness, grief or dysfunctional relationships. Great Horizontal allows us to draw on the strength of a positive foundation in order to eliminate this energy of pain. Connecting to this Energy Release Point brings to awareness the knowledge that the support was always there, for its basis is a Divine Source. It is recognizing that the pain obscured the view. This obscurity is often caused by a dysfunctional relationship to the father or masculine. Through Great Horizontal, one connects to a place where a higher and broader perspective is shown. A place where one can view the horizon at all angles and move in any direction free from past encumbrances brought on by pain and grief. Unblocking and activating this Energy Release Point strengthens the ability to let go of grief in order to make room for vitality. It strengthens the feelings of being supported and loved as well as allows for the development of trust in the masculine.

Disharmonies: *Exhaustion and fatigue; sadness; weeping; sighing; resigned sacrifice of one's own needs for the fulfillment of others; too tired to go on.*

SP-16 Abdomen Sorrow and Lament

Virtues: This Energy Release Point connects into the depths where one finds peace and calm. This is extremely beneficial when life presents experiences of great sorrow such as the loss of a loved one or the loss of a relationship. It allows one to lament and have a passionate expression of grief. It brings compassion and tenderness in times of devastating pain in order to move through distress by flowing tears. Tears must express in order to heal sorrow. Tears serve as a harmonizer and heart balancer. They allow the passage of sorrow so that other emotions can flow in and be experienced. Abdomen Sorrow and Lament is also beneficial for resolution when one feels that they have missed or lost an opportunity. It assists in helping one to release regret and longing for another chance to express what needed to be said in order to find resolution within. Unblocking and activating this Energy Release Point assists in healing the sorrow and distresses in life. It allows for the full expression of distress and emotional pain. It brings a renewal of compassion for Self, strengthens the belief that life continues and that one can trust that needs will once again be met. Through inner peace and calm, connection with spiritual beings and the Divine Source is more easily accessed strengthening the awareness that healing love flows eternal.

Disharmonies: *Deep emotional pain and devastation; grief; longing; loneliness; sorrow; deep seated abandonment and depression; emotional emptiness; inability to see visions of the future thereby blocking creativity and forward motion. Physical manifestations of emotional pain showing as noisy intestines; anxiety; infertility; eating disorders; wasting diseases; weeping body showing as diarrhea.*

SP-17 Food Drain / Destiny Pass

Virtues: This Energy Release Point brings consciousness in regards to one's relationship with food. It gives value to nourishment. It is the awareness and understanding that the Earth Feeds us with her bounty. The care of the Earth facilitates nourishment and the subsequent care of harvesting, preparing and service of food constitutes sacred action. Food that is prepared and served with consciousness and blessed with gratitude before consumption provides an exponential benefit of wholesome nutrients. In early civilizations, the task of gathering and hunting food were regarded as acts of sacredness. It was understood that the Earth was to be treated with reverence and gratitude for its abundance. It was considered an honour to be chosen as a hunter. The hunter understood that animals would seek him knowing that in the next lifetime both would switch places - the hunter becoming the hunted. The hunter therefore demonstrated great awareness and ability in bringing in the prey. Great care would be taken to show mercy to the animal by acting swiftly. Prayers would be offered for a smooth transition and before the fatal cut, the hunter would breath into the mouth of the animal, ensuring the sharing and transferring of his Essence for the next incarnation. Every part of the animal would be used for the benefit of the community and survival. Nothing was wasted. Only the strong and healthy would prepare the food for the community, ensuring the continual health and strength of the people. Gratitude and dances of celebration to the Creator Source would follow, ensuring the success of hunts to come. Understanding sacredness of food extends to conscious eating. Conscious eating and care for the body temple anchors health and well being. This conscious awareness encompasses the absorption of nourishment from life experiences by our Essence. Unblocking and activating this Energy Release Point brings conscious awareness, value and sacredness to food. It empowers the absorption of nutrients for the benefit of life enrichment and wholeness. It assists in learning from life experience, absorbing the beneficial aspects and releasing the inessentials. It strengthens the resolve in viewing ourselves, all of humanity, the vegetable kingdom, the animal kingdom and the Earth as sacred. It brings the awareness and consciousness to the interconnectivity of all and human-ity's role as stewards of the Earth. As the name Destiny Pass implies, it opens up the passageway to receive the bountiful harvest so that one may be nourished to fulfill destiny.

Disharmonies: *Dysfunctional relationship with food; unconsciousness eating such as wastefulness, overeating, abstaining from eating, doing several activities while eating, eating too quickly; feelings of unworthiness; feelings of scarcity and lack; inability to process life experiences efficiently; stuck in a loop of inaction while simultaneously seeking life purpose without follow through on promptings.*

SP-18 Heavenly Stream

Virtues: This Energy Release Point connects one to the Heavenly Stream of the Holy Spirit, an energy transmission of Cosmic Love to the I AM Presence within. It serves to improve the flow of kindness from one to another as one accesses the memory of the truth of who we are - the embodiment of Sacred Essence. This recognition and connection to Essence allows for a further exploration of potential, and through the expression of one's potential, one finds peace, joy and love. In addition, Heavenly Stream empowers empathy and compassion. It allows for a bal-anced flow of reciprocity from within a strong centred consciousness of healthy boundaries. Unblocking and activating this Energy Release Point connects one to their Sacred Essence, allowing for the exploration of potential. In this way, the ability to give nurturing, compassionate care to others comes from a strong self-contained auric field. A field which exudes peace, compassion and healing light.

Disharmonies: *Emotional wounding from feelings of abandonment; misdi-rected love forces which result in dysfunctional merging by over extension of nurturing forces; co-dependence; "Doormat" syndrome from the belief that one receives love only by disempowerment and self-deprecation in servile attitude.*

SP-19 Chest Village

Virtues: This Energy Release Point opens up to the love and compassion of the heart. It empowers the ability to joyfully walk through life. This Energy Release Point is deeply connected to one's relationship to mother and the feminine aspects within. Its location is on the chest, the place where one first bonds with the scent, feel and touch of mother outside of the womb. This is a place where one receives milk and comforting care, connects to the beating of the heart and breathes in heavenly inspiration through the lungs. Chest Village speaks to the birthplace, our special home, nurtured by mother. It is the safe haven where the body connects with the Soul to unearth the passion of potential and the Cord of Life in order to fully participate in life. Unblocking and activating this Energy Release Point connects us to our home, the true home found within our heart of inner truth and wisdom. It allows one to feel empathy for the human condition and move into unconditional love.

Disharmonies: *Dysfunctional relationship with mother; dysfunctional relationship with feminine aspects of Self; inability to feel nurtured and protected; detachment from mothering instincts; being in sympathy; creation of co-dependent relationships.*

SP-20 Encircling Glory

Virtues: This Energy Release Point creates balance between physical and spiritual nourishment, bringing qualities of wholeness and completeness to one's Being. When one is whole and complete, one flourishes. One attracts abundance, joy and health. Wholeness radiates and serves to attract others who are also whole and complete. It is through the virtues of wholeness that one can flourish. Within the energy of wholeness, one finds the energy of loyalty and devotion to the Divine, the Source of ALL. Connecting to Source connects one to purpose and therefore, to joyous service. This is heart centred loyalty and devotion. Unblocking and activating this Energy Release Point allows for the gentle weaving and strengthening of the delicate balance which exists between loyalty to the

Divine, loyalty to the highest good of the Self, as well as that of relation-ships- be it friends, spouse, intimate partner or family member. It balances and harmonizes these relationships to that of our life principles and ideals. It is the balance of altruism in relationship to our connection with others. This delicate balance is strengthened by the Cosmic Law of Reciprocity. To Give and To Receive. It is to integrate the highest level of ourselves, through our loyalty and devotion to the Divine through acts of service which serve to address the needs of others, and in return, receive energy which enriches our wholeness.

Disharmonies: *Neediness; manipulative behaviour; lack of fulfill-ment leading to compulsive grasping; unquenchable desires; the need for instant gratification.*

SP- 21 Great Enveloping

Virtues: This Energy Release Point supports the great embrace of the Divine Feminine and maternal consciousness, much as a womb enfolds the preciousness of the unborn child. It helps distribute this beautiful energy throughout the body as well as bringing energy to nourish the Heart. It reminds one that in order to take care of everyone, one must also take care of oneself. Unblocking and activating this Energy Release Point promotes a return to childlike innocence and trust. It activates self care and allows one to feel loved and nurtured. The return of these feelings allow for a transformational shift to the experience of living and being unconditional love. In this new perception of love, one views humanity with unity consciousness, thus promoting the ability to live in security, so that one can fully embrace life, humanity and the world.

Disharmonies: *Selfishness expressed as neglect for one's own needs; feelings of abandonment and insecurity, especially from the mother; insecurity; dis-trust; isolation; withdrawal from life; pain in the body and joint flaccidity.*

Portraits of the Energy Release Points for the Energy Release Channel of the Heart

HT-1 Utmost Source - to Reach ALL

Virtues: This Energy Release Point connects to the source of ALL THAT IS, aligning the human heart with the Heart of the Divine Source, the Creative Force. It empowers compassion and emotional warmth. It brings the realization of the sacredness of the One and our relationship within the context of being a Divine creation. Unblocking and activating this Energy Release Point strengthens alignment. When in alignment, the realization is that Heaven exists inside one's Being, facilitating the ability to attune to living ones divine expression.

Disharmonies: *Isolation; depression; anxiety; lack of compassion; struggle; chaos and spiritual emptiness.*

HT-2 Blue-Green Vibrancy of Spirit

Virtues: The metaphorical symbology of this Energy Release Point is one of plants growing abundantly over and around an alchemical furnace that is fuelled with Cinnabar. It represents the colour of life, the vibrancy of growth, resurrection, everlasting, freshness, vitality and immortality. Cinnabar is an ancient word derived from the Eastern Indian word for Dragon's blood. The dragon is a representative of the primal forces of Nature and the Universe. It is also associated with wisdom and longevity, possessing great powers of magic. Dragon's blood is highly potent with beneficial qualities of invincibility and protective armour. However, mis-use of the Dragon's blood can lead to death. The qualities of the Cinnabar gemstone stimulates dignity, vitality and power bringing invincibility to the user as it embodies the essence of Dragon's blood. Further imagery is that of alchemical transformation and generative power of growth and transformation. This is evidenced, for example, in the revival of the Earth in spring after a cold and dormant Winter season. Within this symbology is the use of the colour blue-green (Cyan) which represents the colour of growth as embodied by the awakening energy of Spring. Unblocking and activating this Energy Release Point brings transcendence to immortality. It helps one to realize full embodiment of the I AM Presence. It brings composure and reverence that is unaffected by external chaos and turmoil. In this place of power, conscious manifestation of purpose and destiny through ritual is realized. Through conscious creation, life becomes purposeful and conscious living creates conscious leadership. Furthermore, unblocking and activating this Energy Release Point also assists in vanquishing fear and outer terrors, demonic forces and negative entities. Deep awareness of Divine Grace flows into the Heart and through the power of love, forgiveness and compassion, karma is shifted and released.

Disharmonies: *Stuttering; generalized fear as well as fear of transformation and change; heart palpitations; anxiety; insomnia; fear of death.*

HT-3 Little Inner Sea / Lesser Sea

Virtues: This Energy Release Point nourishes the heart and calms the mind from the internal generalized pressure originating from repressed desires or unfulfilled desires. It brings wisdom, depth, peace and inner tranquility. Unblocking and activating this Energy Release Point assists in creating the space and circumstances that allow for great things to come together, bringing to fruition and unlimitedness the manifestation of desires with utmost simplicity.

Disharmonies: *Feelings of being scattered; impatience; anger; frustration; perfectionism especially when the mind is engaged in obsessive thinking without bringing action to plans and vision; inability to move forward toward change; wanting; feeling lack; feeling the oppression of limitation; restriction; oppression.*

HT-4 Path of Spirit

Virtues: This Energy Release point connects one to the philosophy of ancient cultures whose tenets of truth are that the cause of all disease is attributed to the individual not living their purpose and destiny; that disease is the inability to connect to and follow the Path. Healing manifests when one begins to find the Way. The WAY - as exemplified in the ancient document the I-Ching (The Way of Life) or as exemplified by Jesus who said "There are many paths but only one Way". As we raise our vibrations through our evolution to One-ness and Unconditional Love, we resonate closer and closer to the Ascended Masters, Yogi Saints, Christian Saints and other Beings in the Celestial Hierarchy. We do this because we choose the path to enLIGHTenment. We develop the virtues of peace, harmony, joy, wisdom and ONE-ness within ourselves and our world. We draw to us others who are also on the same path to the Way of the LIGHT. Unblocking and activating this Energy Release Point empowers open-ness, receptivity, integrity and righteousness by connecting our Heart and Essence to its spiritual path. It assists in transcendence from the mundane and reconnects to our inner wisdom as defined by our values and our con-science, and the influence of this in the development of our character.

Disharmonies: *Isolation from purpose, overly concerned with the "I" or EGO; attachment to negative ego desires; self-absorbed; self-righteous behaviour; pain and bitterness; betrayal issues.*

HT-5 Penetrating the Interior / Return to Home

Virtues: This Energy Release Point assists in clearing the pathway to Higher Consciousness as we strive to be in One-ness. It brings mental discipline and fuels the intellect. The alternate name Return to Home, shows the ability to integrate the mind/intellect with Spirit, and subsequently direct this integrated awareness internally. Penetrating inwards and returning through conscious awareness in a way which is free and clear of obstruction. It is a return to wholeness, emphasizing harmony within the natural order and Universal Laws. Penetrating the Interior/Return to Home is likened to shining a light within in order to bring insight and understanding to the meaning of life and our place in it. Unblocking and activating this Energy Release Point connects and communicates reason, logic and Cosmic Intellect. When one understands and harmonizes to the Universal Laws, then all things can be created and made manifest.

Disharmonies: *Separation; inability to acknowledge truth; external seeking for the meaning of life; confusion; masking as a form of self-protection; close heartedness; superficial joy; joylessness; suffering in silence and intimacy issues.*

HT-6 Communication Pass / Stone Palace / Penetrating Gate

Virtues: This Energy Release Point speaks to the internal feminine energy, which is cloudy, private and mysterious. It is in the mists. It could be seen as secret, veiled or dark. However, this energy needs to flow unobstructed in order to communicate in a fluent and open manner. Unblocking and activating this Energy Release Point helps make conscious what is unconscious. It releases stuck emotions which hinder the understanding and knowing of who we are. It operates as a light which shines through a crack in the wall of the Stone Palace. The alternate name, Stone Palace is a metaphor of the residence of our Heart, the stones being the walls of the fortress which barricade us from ourselves and from others. Connection with this Energy Release Point allows the Light to create an opening of the gate, a gate which penetrates and accesses the self love of our authentic Being.

Disharmonies: *Hungry heart; over indulgences (in sex, food or drink) in our search for joy and fulfillment; bitterness and pain.*

HT-7 Spirit Gate / Spirit Door / Soul Gate

Virtues: This Energy Release Point connects with the intentions of the Soul through the movement of Spirit within the passageway of the Heart. It allows the Spirit to travel freely with safe passage; to come and go, knowing that it has a place to rest within the home of the Heart. This movement and connection to the intentions of the Soul is about raising the frequency and vibration of our human form. It empowers consciousness to evolve into Mastery. Unblocking and activating this Energy Release Point accesses our ability to empower ourselves to hold our vibration in a stable and centred way. It creates tranquility, peace and heightened devotion to the Oneness. The Soul is always whole and complete and our connection to it through the movement of Spirit makes available to us our deepest source and well-spring for healing.

Disharmonies: *Over-dependance on externals for sources of healing; over-dependence and/or addiction to drugs to inflate or create spiritual experiences; manic/depressive behaviours; mental instability; feelings of being scattered and/or agitated.*

HT-8 Inner Treasures of the Lesser Palace

Virtues: This Energy Release Point speaks metaphorically of the Palace as being the sacred temple of the Divine Self. The Lesser Palace is not smaller or less important, it is the inner chamber of the Heart. It is the place where one can sit in calmness and tranquility in order to reflect on the radiant inner light found there. This is connection to a place within, which calms the Heart and Spirit and brings inner tranquility. Within the space of tranquility, vision can be purified with Spirit and subsequently integrated with the uniqueness of the special gifts that each individual brings to the world. Unblocking and activating this Energy Release Point nurtures the virtues of humility, self worth, and self-assurance. Actions are then expressed in quietness and in gentle revelation. Through this quiet contemplative place, insightful vision of destiny comes effortlessly and Soul expression manifests with ease and grace.

Disharmonies: *Being unreceptive to inner soul promptings; inability to meditate or cultivate inner tranquility; feelings of disconnect; obsessive need to be in control; suppression of self-expression; rage; lack of joy; "burn out" syndrome from over-striving.*

HT-9 Little Thoroughfare

Virtues: This Energy Release Point is the connection to passion and vision. It brings the energy of benevolence and empowers the integration of decision making and planning with the love forces of the Heart. Unblocking and activating this Energy Release Point inspires hope. It develops the ability to trust in the most benevolent outcome and strengthens the intuition. The connection to inner knowing is enhanced and actions that are in alignment with the directives of the heart become the natural response to living.

Disharmonies: *Loss of vision; disconnection with purpose; indecision; hopelessness; hidden fears; nightmares.*

Portraits of the Energy Release Points for the Energy Release Channel of the Small Intestine

SI-1 Little Marsh / Little Happiness

Virtues: This Energy Release Point brings to mind the image of a marsh. A marsh is characterized as being a watery low lying area. It is a geographical place that characteristically shows stagnation and pooling. It collects debris and vegetation from the surrounding environment. This ecosystem however, has vast nutrient value and through sifting and sorting, one can extract the pure essential quality. This purity of substance can then be used to bring beneficial nutrients to other areas of the environment. Unblocking and activating this Energy Release Point brings clarity of thought through the sifting and sorting process. It enhances organizational skills and flexibility within defined structure. This provides great benefit to all aspects of Being. The transformational qualities are alchemical. It is to be able to abstract the purity of truth from the bombardment of information and over stimulation. This is especially important in this time of rapid growth of technology in the modern life experience. The alternate name Little Happiness speaks to the resulting emotion when life is balanced and flowing within organized structure. It is to feel the empowerment which discernment of quality over quantity brings as well as the beneficial effects on the mind when one allows for information to streamline.

Disharmonies: *Mental fuzziness; auto-immune disorders; oversensitivity to environmental toxins; electro-magnetic frequencies; radiation; microwave frequencies; computer emissions and interruptions to the bio-sphere of the human being. There can be repetition of toxic and negative patterning; judgmental attitudes; negativity; inability to follow through on good intentions; inactivity; inability to manifest goals leading to stagnation; sarcasm; cynicism; dysfunctional communication especially in the misinterpretation of truth or the spoken word.*

SI- 2 Forward Valley

Virtues: This Energy Release Point brings us into the valley, a phase of the journey which one must enter and move through in order to reach the destination. A valley is characterized by a darkness that through the movement of the sun brings clarity to the shadows. Unblocking and activating this Energy Release Point empowers the exploration of shadows by bringing light into the depths. It empowers the ability to know the true self through introspection, insight, intuition, and inner guidance. It encourages deep listening. Listening to the inner recesses of the Heart which convey messages from deep within. The clarity of light ensures the ability to receive these messages and therefore accurately communicate these heart messages to the world.

Disharmonies: *Sarcasm; bitterness; disconnection from Heart essence (purpose and destiny) leading to looking externally for the causes of pain; seeking guidance outside one's knowing leading to confusion, control issues, and creation of a false persona/or stories about who we are and how life is; conflicts and fear between desires, commitment and need; manifestation of bladder infections; fear and separation.*

SI-3 Back Ravine

Virtues: This Energy Release Point brings the flexibility needed to overcome obstacles which block one from staying on their course. There are many paths to connection to soul purpose and vision, and regardless of which path we choose, the goal is to arrive at the final destination. Back Ravine brings flexibility to the process and assists in the navigation of life. It strengthens inter-dependence and clarity, allowing for the discernment to know how, and when, to ask for assistance in order to create situations of positive outcome. It strengthens trust in the Divine plan. Unblocking and activating this Energy Release Point empowers trust. A trust that comes from the connection to our inner wisdom and intuition. A trust that evolves from the practice of discernment and alignment to Truth. As one re-connects with Soul Purpose, the natural outcome is that the physical body benefits by being nourished from within. Back Ravine builds strong forces of vital energy, by generating the continual flow of trust when walking the path.

Disharmonies: *Lack of clarity; untapped forces of masculine forthrightness; lack of vitality.*

SI-4 Wrist Bone

Virtues: This Energy Release Point is seen both metaphorically and physically as the junction between our core self and our extension into the world. It is to extend ourselves and make contact with others through the social process. By extending ourselves we can convey our heart's message into the world. It is to extend ourselves to be of service to humanity through the dissemination of our gifts. When this Energy Release Point is free flowing, our heart's message is directed through our speech and positive action as well as embodying the Law of Reciprocity. That is: to give and to receive. Unblocking and activating this Energy Release Point helps us to reach out into the world so that we can receive what we need to nourish our Essence. Thus, we walk through life with trust, commitment to our inner purpose and conscience, with assurance and confidence to complete our tasks.

Disharmonies: *Self doubt; mistrust; bitterness; sarcasm and cynicism.*

SI-5 Sun Warmed Valley

Virtues: This Energy Release Point brings one to a place of fertility, regeneration and growth. Connecting with this Sun Warmed Valley allows for the Solar Energy to come in and provide a catalytic spark. A spark which serves to enrich and activate the fecundity of the Valley in order for it to reach its full potential. This Energy Release Point has a modulating effect which balances the qualities of heart's passion, desire, Divine Will and Spiritualized Ego with the little will and negative ego. This Sun Warmed Valley allows for the reception of Light as well as for the understanding of the Divine encoded messages which are embedded in this Light. This Light comes from the Heart and Pulse of the Universal ALL, therefore it is based on the frequencies of Cosmic Love. These Love based messages bring the clarity necessary to distinguish that which is of higher aspiration from that which are negative ego wants and needs. This allows for the process of the release of the extraneous while holding onto wisdom. Unblocking and activating this Energy Release Point brings an elevation of conscious awareness that allows the sparks of sun fire to illuminate and fuel the action of the will to align with higher Divine Will. This catalytic spark nourishes the fruition of desires and brings into manifestation the integration of coherent thinking, speech and action with higher Soul functions.

Disharmonies: *Weak willed; inability to cope; hopelessness; stagnation in action; lack of fulfillment; distorted sense of self; ego inflation or self-effacement; ego driven and over concern with the physical; fanaticism; mania; delusions with reality.*

SI-6 Nourishing the Old

Virtues: This Energy Release Point has the ability to nourish the Emotional Body when facing and healing pain from the past. Oftentimes, events of the present can trigger memories of traumatic and painful events of the past. Pain that was buried and unaddressed creating stagnation and heaviness in the physical body. Unblocking and activating this Energy Release Point empowers the assimilation of life's lessons, bringing forward the jewel of learning from having experienced these traumas. It breaks the cycle of negativity and releases the energy of victim. It quells and transforms suffering into blessings of peace and gratitude. Stagnation is released and brings revitalizing energy to all levels of the body - the physical, emotional, mental and spiritual aspects by clearing the congestion of one's perception of life. From elevated consciousness, one may more easily feel the passion of destiny and purpose.

Disharmonies: *Lethargy; weakness; pain or paralysis of the arms and legs; overwhelm and confusion; manifestation of cynicism; bitterness and sarcasm due to oppression by only seeing the worst in everything; confusion due to our past noxiously colouring the present - affecting our ability to interpret life experiences accurately in a positive way; negative interpretations of life.*

SI-7 Support Uprightness

Virtues: This Energy Release Point clears the mind through releasing inner stagnation. It re-establishes the clarity of the message from the Heart, to its faithful communication to the outside world. It strengthens the physical body, in particular the limbs, to convey the heart's intention to the world with accuracy. Unblocking and activating this Energy Release Point empowers clarity and intuition. It is to know the world directly with our heart by connecting with our higher self and I AM Presence. It is to stand upright, between heaven and earth and perceive life without judgement. It conveys the heart's purpose and intentions into the world through both speech and action, bridging clear communication and virtuous deeds.

Disharmonies: *Sarcasm; bitterness; actions that perpetuate our own suffering and suffering of others; confusion.*

SI-8 Small Sea

Virtues: This Energy Release Point balances the relationship between sorting and transformation, during threshold experiences when one must evaluate and discern. It accesses and relates to conscious awareness the lessons learned from life experiences so that one can let go and move into a place of more awareness. In this way, one can release trauma and pain from the body in a conscious way. Unblocking and activating this Energy Release Point provides the awareness and healing of painful experiences. It brings a movement of energy to disintegrate the blocks which have hindered the soul's ability to fully experience full, grounded embodiment. The gift of embodiment is to fully participate in the process of life. Incarnation in of itself, serves as a foundation and centre of containment of the soul expression. Small Sea activates the true expression of alchemy between the passionate fire of Masculine forces and the watery sources of the Feminine forces in order to activate and embrace life purpose.

Disharmonies: *Confusion; slowed thought processes; having the impression of working hard to earn a living but never enjoying the fruits of labor;*

sadness; bitterness; failure to be nourished by life experiences in all aspects of being.

SI - 9 Upright Shoulder / Shoulder Integrity / True Shoulder

Virtues: This Energy Release Point empowers the virtues of integrity and the inner moral compass of righteousness so that one stands in clarity and acts decisively in one's right action. It allows one to embrace life with renewed enthusiasm, fervour and active engagement in community and world events. In Ancient China, the scapula of the shoulder was often used in divination to foresee good fortune and luck. It was understood that if one stood in uprightness of character and walked their path in virtue, good luck and fortune would always follow. Therefore, this Energy Release Point speaks to responsibility, that is, the responsibility we hold within ourselves to the appropriate response to what we know as truths. To devote ourselves to the recognition and the understanding of the Truth - then to be firmly devoted to this truth in the same way as we honour the I AM Presence within. Unblocking and activating this Energy Release Point helps one to stand in his/her truth. A truth that is pure and in integrity and alignment with right action. In this energy, one is incorruptible and far less likely to veer off the path of purpose and destiny.

Disharmonies: *Extremes of fanaticism or apathy; self-righteousness or self-deprecation; anger over injustices or stagnation of action. Physically this can show as pain and inflammation in the shoulder.*

SI-10 Shoulder Blade

Virtues: This Energy Release Point is named for it's geographical location of the shoulder blade. It is the meeting point of the Energy Release Channel of the Small Intestine, the Extraordinary Energy Release Channel of the Masculine Vessel of Movement and the Extraordinary Energy Release Channel of the Masculine Vessel of Structure. The resulting benefit of this Energy Release Point therefore speaks to the creation of an energy which is greater than the sum of its parts. It is the ability to shoulder the responsibilities of life and helps one to stand in a strong and erect manner. It is stability and centre and as such, keeps everything in balance, nourishing the health of the physical body. It opens a conduit which flows a dynamic source of vitality. It serves to circulate this vitality through the body so that one successfully accomplishes one's mission, reminding us that the Soul is immortal and we are here to share our gifts in service to the elevation of consciousness of humanity. Unblocking and activating this Energy Release Point increases life energy so that one can encounter situations with confidence. It assists in balancing one's unique individuality with the energy of group consciousness so that one can function in wholeness within a larger social matrix.

Disharmonies: *Blocks the free flow of energy of the Secondary Energy Centre of the shoulder.*

SI-11 Celestial Gathering / Heavenly Assembly of the Ancestors

Virtues: This Energy Release Point has strong roots in creation mythologies. Physically this point is located on the scapula - the shoulder blade; where one can visualize the unfurling of angel wings. All of humanity shares creation mythology - one creation with many variants of the story. The basis of these myths is the common thread that we were once ONE with the Creator - The ALL - the Universal Source - the Creative Force. The Creator set about the task of creation of the world over a span of time. In this time, the polarities of which we are all familiar were created. The sky separated from the Earth, the clouds separated from the oceans, light separated from darkness, humanity separated from the vastness of the ALL and man created separation from woman. These creations of polarity not only manifested in the physical world, but also represent an event in the Universal Mind. That is: Heart separated from Mind - the universal to the individual and the macrocosm to the microcosm. All this is done with the goal to create individual consciousness and make the development of the EGO SELF possible. By unblocking and activating this Energy Release Point, we are reminded that we are part of a wholeness; the Creative Force; the ALL - although separate by nature of our individual physicality.

This realization in itself brings a state of mental repose and tranquility. Unblocking and activating this point brings about a state of calmness. Through inner tranquility, realization comes that one is not alone in human suffering. It is this perception and awareness that humanity has a shared experience and therefore, resolving our own dilemmas drawn from the wisdom of those who have gone before us is facilitated. Depth of insight brings understanding, peace and inspiration. Unblocking and activating this Energy Release Point also allows for insight into the wisdom of our elders - our lineage, and those who have passed. Acknowledging and honouring the past, as well as that of our lineage, followed by integration of the jewels of learning, brings greater fulfillment and abundance within our co-creative acts as we move through life. Connecting to our ancestry allows us to open and to be guided by innate wisdom which may present as dreams. These dreams help us access the vision of our Soul, as well as the dreams of the Ancestor Consciousness, and make peace with being human, accept our limitations and our inability to completely know and comprehend life. Thus, to surrender.

Disharmonies: *Separation anxiety; feelings of malaise; inability to let go; control issues; overwhelm and disorganization; feelings of separation from family; alienation.*

SI-12 Grasping the Wind

Virtues: This Energy Release Point releases hypersensitivity and over-stimulation that confuses the ability to sort, discern and distinguish. Unblocking and activating this Energy Release Point promotes mental clarity by harmonizing the processes of decision making and organizing. It restores calm from chaos. (Chaos which shifts the energy field creating the feeling of being ungrounded.) As a Wind Entry Point, it is an access point for pernicious energies; especially those energies of fear which the wind sweeps from the planet. This Energy Release Point supports the energy of seriousness and commitment towards a directed life purpose and vocation.

Disharmonies: *Poor decision making; chaotic thoughts; physically one can feel shoulder stiffness and pain; inflammation and limited range of motion; racing thoughts and speech leading to incoherency.*

SI-13 Crooked Wall

Virtues: This Energy Release Point has the interesting name of Crooked Wall. Crooked can bring to mind that which has strayed from convention or has strayed from alignment to integrity. Walls are boundaries; both physical and energetic. In one sense, the physical body has a defined immune system which protects the physical body from external forces of invasion. However the strength of the immune system correlates to the strength of the alignment to purpose and integrity. When one is bent - that is not congruent with one's Self - there are distortions between the heart and physical action. This is often the main cause of body disharmony leading to disease. Emotional, mental and spiritual immunity is then compromised and one may become weak, fearful and obsessive. This breakdown of the body defences further leads to the susceptibility of invasion of psychic astral entities which leads to further fracturing and parasitic influence. This Energy Release Point strengthens and protects all aspects of the immune system by helping one to re-align with the integrity of their higher self.

Disharmonies: *Deceptive behaviour; denial; dishonesty; estrangement from higher spiritual authority and inner wisdom; nervous fear and obsessive compulsive behaviours; paranoia; low vitality and energy leading to sickness and disease.*

SI-14 Outside the Shoulder

Virtues: This Energy Release Point is named for its geographical location on the body. As a shoulder point it serves to release pain of the shoulder and increase the shoulder's range of motion. When unblocking and activating this Energy Release Point, one should question as to the cause of the block of energy flow. This cause is diverse; for some, it is over responsibility, for others, it is a question of boundaries and either taking on, or shouldering the loads which belong to others. The cause of the blockage is usually from an external condition and it serves as a reminder to go inside and question why we sacrifice.

Disharmonies: *Weariness and fatigue; having the feeling of burden and irksome duty; pain in the shoulder; limited range of motion.*

SI-15 Middle of the Shoulder

Virtues: This Energy Release Point allows for suppleness and flexibility in mind, body and spirit. It empowers one to see the bigger picture so that one can practice "the middle way". It helps in achieving moderation and balance. Unblocking and activating this Energy Release Point allows one to access the perspective of a greater overview. From this heightened state of awareness, one can more easily see the expansion of many possibilities and unlimited potential.

Disharmonies: *Pain in the body; rigidity in the body; rigidity of the mind; inflexibility in all aspects of being; narrow scope of consciousness.*

SI-16 Window Cage / Window of Heavenly Brightness

Virtues: This Energy Release Point assists in opening up to clear and pure vision of our inner core. This is especially beneficial when we want to see beyond our ordinary existence and connect to the beauty both within ourselves and our outer world. When this Energy Release Point is unblocked and activated, it creates a gradual illumination. An illumination which strengthens in magnitude as we begin to see, focus and contemplate the beauty surrounding us. As we develop our senses from this place of awareness, we can more appreciate, with awe, the spirit of nature as it unfolds and reveals it's wonders. This process empowers from within the virtues of gratitude, beauty and joy. As reference to it's name being that of a window - it reminds us that a window can open and close according to our interpretation of life experiences. Choosing to keep the window open, we can see life events from a clear perspective and are encouraged to receive wisdom to release patterns of suffering; suffering which can manifest as toxins in the physical body.

Disharmonies: *Cynicism; bitterness; seeing the negative in every person, place or situation; mistrust as to the intentions of others; to be suspicious; inability to connect with love of self, love of life, or love of others in a full-hearted, embracing way.*

SI-17 Heavenly Appearance

Virtues: This Energy Release Point carries the theme of connection. Connection with the Higher Aspects of Self and ultimately connection with the Divine Self. In order for this connection to happen, one must look to see the bigger picture and have a shift in perspective. Unblocking and activating this Energy Release Point creates a shift in perspective, a shift which promotes a purification energy. Heavenly Appearance casts light on negativity and burns away suffering.

Disharmonies: *Feeling isolated; lack of joy; narrow scope of consciousness.*

SI-18 Cheekbone Hole / Influential Bone Hole

Virtues: This Energy Release Point brings to consciousness the observation that the strength of the cheekbone is a reflection of the strength of the bones of the whole body. The strength of the bones is also a reflection of Body alignment with the Heart's passion. The strength of the cheekbone therefore is determined by one's ability to convey the Heart's Essence through one's speech. This Energy Release Point assists in connecting and expressing the fire of the Soul as nourished by the Heart in it's altruism and inner ideals. This joy-filled passion can then nourish, inspire and encourage others.

Disharmonies: *Willful influence on others; distorted ego self; inability to communicate spiritual ideals. Physically one may experience symptoms of pain and tension in the jaw.*

SI-19 Listening Palace

Virtues: This Energy Release Point empowers listening with your spirit, for spirit is existential emptiness and therefore open to receive. It develops and cultivates intuition. It restores the ability to communicate clearly by integrating the virtues of feminine receptive listening and forthright masculine seeing. Unblocking and activating this Energy Release Point brings greater conscious awareness to the communicator. It stimulates attentive listening in order to actively receive the pearls of wisdom from our Ascended Master teachers. One must be attentive in order to hear with the Heart and therefore, Listening Palace assists in purifying and cleansing our Heart. The ear becomes the vehicle for the reception of truth.

Disharmonies: *Inability to meditate or pray; lack of attuning to soul insight; disorganized communication; lack of focus and concentration.*

Portraits of the Energy Release Points for the Energy Release Channel of the Urinary Bladder

UB-1 Eyes Full of Illumination

Virtues: This Energy Release Point assists us in discerning the difference between looking and seeing. It opens up the mind's eye and the spiritual eye in order to form clear perceptions of reality, free from judgment and limitation. When one begins to observe what is around them, then one can begin to describe what is seen. This strengthens the ability to be present, really beginning to see and observe for the first time, and then, beginning to see more and more. The wise one will begin to observe and describe the beauty of what is seen. Therefore, the more one sees, connects and holds the description of beauty in the mind's eye - the more the eyes will open with wonder and awe. The eyes begin to fill with illuminated consciousness to see the radiance of the Creative Force in all things. Unblocking and activating this Energy Release Point allows our eyes to open and be filled with the brightness of Spirit. It allows for the alchemy of transforming our vision through the insights and connection to the Spiritual Alchemist's work of creating a golden elixir. It is illumination, compassion and radiance. It brings clarity and wisdom into perfect balance. From this, we are energized and more capable of greeting each day with enthusiasm and vitality.

Disharmonies: *Misperception of reality; distortions of truth; fear; depression.*

UB-2 The Grasping of Bamboo / Origin Pillar

Virtues: This Energy Release Point speaks to the metaphor of bamboo and it's representation of virtue. The bamboo plant is made of segments that fit into each other in an orderly, strong way. However, the leaves arch gracefully from the trunk which is hollow. In heavy storms, the entire plant is flexible, stays rooted into the earth and is seldom broken. It's ability to withstand great winds in combination with it's other qualities allows for it to be harmonious with it's environment. It's strength allows for it to be a pillar. When one adapts the qualities of bamboo to oneself, it facilitates our ability to be alive and present; experiencing all that embracing life brings. Staying connected with our environment, the earth, nature and the homes that shelter us. To hold true to our foundation or core integrity with the essential awareness of the Abyss or the VOID. The receptive emptiness which allows us to receive the Light of Illumination and Wisdom of our True Self. Dropping away all that is extraneous as well as any chaotic disturbances will lead to deeper states of calmness and equanimity. Connecting with Ultimate Truth having the liberating insight that is free from the grasping tendencies of the mind. Unblocking and activating this Energy Release Point assists in the alignment of oneself with integrity and being willing to admit to the actual motivation behind actions and the actual benefits or harm that these actions may cause. It allows then for the opportunity to create a higher choice for the good of all.

Disharmonies: *Over identification with the illusionary aspects of oneself; creating and living in a dysfunctional and chaotic environment; pettiness; hoarding tendencies; overly concerned with trivial matters.*

UB-3 Eyebrows Rushing

Virtues: This Energy Release Point integrates the idea of viewing from the top or elevated perspective with the idea of the flexibility and the strength of water. The characteristics of flexibility and versatility of water empowers the strength and ability of water to move through and around an obstacle in its path. The image this Energy Release Point evokes is that of standing at the edge of a source of water and feeling the power of an erupting geyser. This Energy Release Point empowers a point of view or perspective of the exciting adventure of life and transforms vitality and versatility of rushing water into enthusiasm and motivation for action. Unblocking and activating this Energy Release Point brings clear vision to see the next steps with brightness and clarity. This brightness empowers the ability to draw on the depths and connect with the great vital force of water and thereby generate momentum and quick action.

Disharmonies: *Obscured vision; overactivity and anxiety due to an overwhelming sense of urgency.*

UB-4 Deviating Servant

Virtues: This Energy Release Point assists in the transformation of knowledge into wisdom. The Energy Release Points for the Energy Release Channel of the Urinary Bladder, beginning with the first, UB-1 Eyes Full of Illumination, ascending to UB-7 Penetrate Heaven, represent the integration of Divine Inspiration and the ability to draw on sources of energy as required to fulfill the physical manifestation of these inspired Divine directives. The fine tuning of this integration is based upon the strength of one's perception of reality and the clarity of the mind. The name Deviating Servant expresses two concepts. The first is that of human tendency to stray from one's goals and purpose, to turn aside or diverge from a course of action. Many instances present and again one finds themselves departing from living one's truth and authenticity. It is the allowing of distractions that bring inconsistency to action, and as a result, brings mental confusion and questioning of what comes next in the plan of life. The second concept is that of servant. The imbalances manifesting as actions taken on behalf of others, again deviating from one's purpose and fulfillment of authentic desires. Unblocking and activating this Energy Release Point harmonizes the servant, that is, it strengthens resolve and the servant becomes the strength to serve for the highest good and benefit of the One. It assists in the ability to connect with inspiration and authentic truth of One's purpose, as well as strengthens the ability to function with clarity and set intention. In this way, acquired experience and knowledge transform into the wisdom of one who can master intentions of the Soul and serve to the benefit of all.

Disharmonies: *Mental fatigue from the overuse of willpower; feeling as though one is floundering; overextending in the effort to achieve goals; inability to reconcile one's perception of reality with life's circumstances; being inconsistent in actions and goals; inability to make up one's mind and make firm decisions or intentions; inability to connect and act upon one's purpose and destiny. Physical manifestation of sinusitis.*

UB-5 Fifth Place

Virtues: This Energy Release Point helps to create a shift in consciousness. The number five is often used to describe the state of perfection, such as the qualities of the fifth dimension. Numerically, five has a very special quality, bringing openings to new beginnings, transformative leaps, the ability to move in a great or impressive way. This Energy Release Point represents change. Change with a ferocity coming from the awakening of Spirit. This transformation, however, comes from a place of centre that is fuelled by the energy of self nurturance. Unblocking and activating this Energy Release Point helps us to connect to the importance of following the laws of nature, such as what we observe in the cycles of the planet. A cycle which balances and nourishes life. Honouring a time to rest, a time to play, a time for the society of others, a time for solitude. Once we embody this cycle, we find harmony and stability, setting the conditions for transformation, strengthening our ability to leap forward free of fear, doubt and uncertainty.

Disharmonies: *Stagnation; fear; anxiety; overwhelm; unclear vision.*

UB-6 Receive Light

Virtues: This Energy Release Point empowers us to accept our responsibilities in a way that is free from anxiety or fear. It allows for an opening that recognizes and receives solar masculine strength which affirms the knowing that one is always supported. When responsibilities are accepted from strength of service of benevolence, fear and anxiety cannot exist. Instead, there is pure illumination and knowledge to take the steps towards freedom from the Universal Law of Cause and Effect. It is to be conscious in the process of evolution that embraces the Universal Law of Accumulated Good. Unblocking and activating this Energy Release Point allows us to recognize our brilliance and awaken to the realization of our potential. It furthers this recognition to take responsibility for our creations and to move forward in service to the benefit of human evolution.

Disharmonies: *Darkness and depression; disconnected from purpose; struggling to act upon what one knows needs to be done; resisting action and avoidance of reality.*

UB-7 Penetrate Heaven / Celestial Connection / Old as the Heavens

Virtues: This Energy Release Point assists in bringing the Energy of Peace where there is trouble and despair, by penetrating through the chaos and connecting with the Firmament of Heaven. The Firmament being the vibratory protective shield of consciousness which surrounds our planet that has been placed there by Celestial Beings of Light. Penetrate Heaven allows us direct access to a higher dimensional consciousness so that calm and peace of mind can ensue. It is the point of consciousness that reminds us that we are linked to, and part of, a higher heavenly consciousness. It is a consciousness that extends itself to be present in every now moment of life. The central function of this Energy Release Point is to link the point of Light within the Mind of God to the point of Light within the minds of humanity so that we may shine our Light through the manifestation of our gifts, talents and intellectual brilliance to the world in service for the world. This point of brilliance also serves to remind us to reach up to Heaven and realize our potential, to move to the highest within us to ultimately reach the God Force in purified virtuous form. Unblocking and activating this Energy Release Point allows us to address the pinnacle of our outer manifestation of our Essence. In the aspect of the name Old as the Heavens, it helps one to connect to the wisdom of the innate gifts and talents that have come to us through the cultivation of virtues by our ancestors. By realizing these virtues and acting on them through wisdom as opposed to fear brought on by chaos, we can heal the needs of the Souls of our ancestors and free ourselves on another level through a deeper understanding of the Universal Law of Cause and Effect.

Disharmonies: *Fear; overwhelm; feelings of disconnection; loneliness and isolation; chaotic lifestyle; unawareness of the Universal Law of Cause and Effect; inability to recognize or develop talents and natural abilities.*

UB-8 Connecting Cleft

Virtues: This Energy Release Point marks the beginning of the downward flow of energy through the Energy Release Channel of the Urinary Bladder. The word cleft means a split or division. This Energy Release Point serves as a bridge of connection to span the separation between the Spiritual Realm and the Physical Realm. It ensures that although we experience a physical form, we are still a spiritual being connected to the ALL That Is. The apex of illumination achieved by UB-7 Penetrate Heaven/Celestial Connection/Old as the Heavens, has the ability to integrate into physicality through Connecting Cleft. This Energy Release Point can then communicate the messages of Light by flowing the stream of Spirit into every aspect of being. These messages of Light are encodements of the Divine Self. Unblocking and activating this Energy Release Point activates self realization. It helps to raise one's vibrational frequency towards a greater connection with the Divine Self in order to flow destiny and purpose.

Disharmonies: *Difficulty choosing a vocation; difficulty in staying on one's spiritual path; unexplained fatigue or weariness; difficulty letting go of habits or attitudes that knowingly create hindrance.*

UB-9 Jade Pillow

Virtues: This Energy Release Point embodies the characteristics of Jade. The preciousness and the beauty. Jade is a stone that assists in the raising of consciousness thereby strengthening the clarity and the ability to discern purpose. It inspires inner peace, intuition and wisdom. The name Jade Pillow, evokes the state of being in which one may rest in the gentle arms of sleep. The rested state facilitates the ability to function within the busy-ness of diverse activities of life. It helps to brighten the eyes for a more keen perception of reality strengthening the ability to navigate circumstances which otherwise can cause stress. Unblocking and activating this Energy Release Point allows for an increase in discernment. It realigns the flowing energy of the two Energy Release Channels of the Divine Feminine Matrix and the Divine Masculine Director, which move energy through the central axis of the body - unifying the three vital energies of Heaven, Humanity and the Earth known as the Three Treasures. Jade is a treasure, the realization of one's precious sacredness and beauty of the Soul. Jade Pillow restores the ability to find the jewel of optimism in all of life's circumstances in order to renew clarity of purpose. As these virtues are enhanced by the unblocking of this Energy Release Point, one receives the gift of grace, comfort and ease knowing that it is acceptable to let go and let God look after the stresses of the day. It activates the law of Divine Grace bringing absolute knowingness that with the Divine - all is possible. With the mind in quiet repose, restful sleep ensues. Rest is then valued as a source of regeneration for all aspects of being.

Disharmonies: *Mental exhaustion, inability to rest and anxiety.*

UB-10 Heavenly Pillar

Virtues: This Energy Release Point connects us to an inner pillar of strength and empowers us to transcend fear. It is the pillar of Spirit that empowers us to hold our heads up and stand tall with renewed self-confidence. It is the clear perception of our abilities and the understanding that we have what it takes to complete our tasks and do our work. Here we come to our central pillar of strength that connects to the core of our Being. Here we know that we have faith in ourselves and that we are supported by the Divine Beings that surround us. Unblocking and activating this Energy Release Point empowers one to stand up for oneself and live one's beliefs free from fear. Additionally it assists in bringing perspective as we move towards aligning with Heavenly directives felt by Soul promptings which, by consequence, increase our physical vitality through acting with the inner wisdom of the heart.

Disharmonies: *Lack of confidence or faith in oneself; feeling unsupported; disempowered; overwhelmed.*

UB-11 Great Shuttle / One Hundred Labours

Virtues: This Energy Release Point assists with clarity and organization of vision. It is one of the first steps to re-vitalize and rejuvenate the physical body. Visualize the shuttle creating a beautiful woven tapestry, a metaphor representing the picture of our lifestream's journey, the intricate threads of detail weaving our life in harmony with the cycles and patterns of nature and in our interactions with others. Life has movement. The shuttle has a beautiful rhythmic movement, an embodiment of the Fifth Universal Principal of Rhythm. This movement creates dynamic patterns that enrich all aspects of our Being as well as co-operatively connecting these aspects so that ALL functions in harmony. The more that we connect and flow with this rhythmic weaving, the more our vitality is enriched with the end result being a healthy, wholesome, rejuvenated life force. The alternate name, One Hundred Labours, alludes to the toll that life can take in depleting us. Unblocking and activating this Energy Release Point assists in melting resistance to taking the necessary steps towards rest and allowing for the rebuilding of strength.

Disharmonies: *Exhaustion; physical collapse; resisting rest.*

UB-12 Gateway of the Winds

Virtues: This Energy Release Point is the gateway to the winds of change. Wind is movement and life is about movement. Movement through the seasons, cycles and year in a continuous forward activity. Gateway of The Winds opens up the portal of energy to expand, fuel and nourish our vitality. A vitality which strengthens and builds both the physical and etheric vitality. This strengthens the ability to distinguish beneficial or non-beneficial energies - seen and unseen- in the environment as well as in social relationships. Unblocking and activating this Energy Release Point accesses the inner tranquility of the heart so that one can connect with the ability to sense and discern the energy of movement. It further helps one to understand why the change is beneficial, as well as accessing the flow of energy required to take the appropriate action towards the change in question.

Disharmonies: *Weakened immune system for both the physical body and astral body; mediumistic tendencies; headaches; nasal disorders; congestions; discharge; sneezing and nosebleeds; coughs.*

UB-13 Lung Connection

Virtues: This Energy Release Point provides a clear connection to inspiration, soul-filled artistry and creativity. It is a connection to the Divine Source. It is a tangible power which impels one to manifest, creating ease in actualization. It is an energy which activates desire born of purpose. It strengthens the willingness to embrace life with enthusiasm. Unblocking and activating this Energy Release Point allows for the full integration of inspiration with the physical vehicle. It helps one stay grounded and focused so that true artistic and creative potential can manifest.

Disharmonies: *Lack of direction; inability to bring creative forces into physical manifestation.*

UB-14 Tower Gate

Virtues: This Energy Release Point speaks to empowered, balanced boundaries. Much as the name implies, it is similar to a lookout tower for the Soul/Spirit/Body. It steadfastly guards one's best interests and empowers feelings of safety and security. Unblocking and activating this Energy Release Point provides connection to a reservoir of strength so that one may stand tall with dignity and honour.

Disharmonies: *Inability to recognize the strength of the Divine Feminine; low self esteem; inability to erect healthy boundaries leading to doormat syndrome; to be weak willed; faint of heart.*

UB-15 Connecting Space of the Heart and Mind

Virtues: This Energy Release Point connects the wisdom, compassion and love of the Sacred Fires of the Heart with the will and intentions of the mind. It facilitates the alignment between the central core of integrity, inner conscience and outward words and actions. It is through commitment to one's inner truths and wisdom of the Heart that one finds the perfection of freedom. Freedom becomes based on the ability to create action and be of service through the sheer joy and love of the service in itself. Freedom in this way is the seed for the basis of fifth dimensional consciousness and way of life. The alchemy of this connection is that it catalyzes the Will and Heart for transformation. In this way it brings versatility, flexibility and adaptability of the Heart/Mind to integrate with the third dimensional physical plane. This alignment of Heart and mind creates a strong reserve of energy. An energy that fuels the heart's passion, strengthens the will and formulates intention so that fulfillment of purpose and destiny actualizes. Unblocking and activating this Energy Release Point creates a space for unity consciousness and fifth dimensional living. It enhances an environment of honour, respect and reverence, for self and others, through the ability to recognize the divine within.

Disharmonies: *Fear leading to heart palpitations, poor memory, anxiety, grief, excessive caution, insomnia, disorientation, excessive dreaming, mania-depression, epilepsy, dementia.*

UB-16 Tower of the Divine Masculine Director / Tower Benefit / Tower Cover

Virtues- This Energy Release Point reinvigorates the full body system by creating a strong interface between the physical, emotional, mental and spiritual bodies, as well as the Energy Body and the Energy Fields. The physical body has many systems, physical and non-physical, which integrate together to create the all round health and well being of an individual. When there has been trauma, chronic illness, or inborn constitution weakness due to genetic lineage, the whole body system may be loosely connected, disjointed or fragmented. This can lead to severe depletion, with the seeming inability to draw on the regenerative self healing forces of the body. Unblocking and activating this Energy Release Point serves to mend together the whole body system. It transforms fear into wisdom, as vital energy recirculates throughout our systems, helping one to ground into physicality and step onto the path with stability and security. It assists one to stand up in all aspects of being so that one's purpose and intentions for life are reclaimed and asserted.

Disharmonies: *Burning the candle at both ends in an effort to keep up with the pace of life and material influences of others; fractured consciousness leading to overwhelm and compromised immunity; prone to entity invasion, thereby not feeling like oneself; the need to impress others by our accomplishments, due to measuring self worth by successes as defined by others; filled with self importance; instability and lack of grounding.*

UB-17 Diaphragm Connection

Virtues- This Energy Release Point gently parts the veil of separation allowing for a glimpse of the higher dimensional consciousness of the seventh dimension. This is a consciousness that embraces compassion, acceptance, forgiveness, deep joy and devotion. It is part of the ascension process where one can perceive and communicate with the Masters, to grasp and understand God-truths. When one has the mastery of the knowledge of God-truth, then illumination is attained. It is to connect and live in a World of Love, where one moves higher yet in vibration, to transcend the knowledge of God-truth to the higher level of Unconditional Love. Unblocking and activating this Energy Release Point allows us to open up the heart, so that when one is ready to embrace a seventh dimensional consciousness it flows into physical manifestation on the earth plane. It is the glimpse of an extraordinary, attainable reality shown to those who are ready to have deep connection within self and consequently with others. It promotes self acceptance, acceptance and tolerance for others, peace and equanimity.

Disharmonies: *Stagnation resulting from conflict - conflict within self or conflict within relationships; feelings of separation and isolation largely due to a painful separation of an intimate relationship.*

UB-18 Ninth Burning Space / Liver Connection

Virtues: This Energy Release Point connects to a place of satisfaction, contentment, peace and inner tranquility. There is a sense of satisfaction of accomplishment and internal recognition that comes from attaining the completion of a project instrumental to the health of the Soul. Within this satisfaction is the awareness that as one places closure on a creative process, the process itself sets the foundation for a new cycle of activity. Unblocking and activating this Energy Release Point provides movement and flow towards new goals inspired by vision and fuelled by contentment. It helps bring forward beginnings. As the name Ninth Burning Space, one also activates the energy of purification needed to release the energies of frustration, anger, depression and judgment in order to move forward towards Soul promptings and live one's destiny.

Disharmonies: *Stress and anxiety; inner turmoil; unrest; non achievement; inability to catalyze will forces to purposeful action; depression; self-judgment; low self-esteem.*

UB-19 Gallbladder Connection

Virtues: This Energy Release Point empowers the virtue of courage. The courage to transform dreams into reality and the courage to overcome obstacles. It addresses the ability to have clear focus aligned with the higher directives of the Soul in regards to vision and purpose. It accesses an energy which provides strength. Unblocking and activating this Energy Release Point allows for the action of synthesis. It brings together the plan and vision of the Soul with the force of courage, clarity and focus.

Disharmonies: *Irritation; stagnation; inability to act; indecisive.*

UB-20 Eleventh Burning Space / Spleen Connection

Virtues: This Energy Release Point is a point of transformation and alchemy. The spleen occupies a vital function in the organ system. It transfers, transports and absorbs nourishment into our full body system. On the physical level, it transforms nutrients into vital energy. On the emotional level, the spleen transforms insight into intuition. On the mental level, the spleen transforms information into knowledge. On the spiritual level, the spleen transforms knowledge into consciousness. This elevated consciousness brings to awareness the strength of aligning with inner truth and realization of one's divinity. All this alchemy has a common goal and that is to transform what is on a basic level towards a higher vibratory level. A higher vibratory level where our thought processes can flow easily, as well as be nourished by life experiences. Unblocking and activating this Energy Release Point allows for alchemy, the energy of burning away remnants of the lower self and move into Spiritual mastery on all planes (physical, emotional, mental and spiritual). It brings an invigoration of energy so that we are better able to present ourselves and our gifts of service to the world, and by so doing, we open to the exchange and therefore are better able to receive, process and integrate the abundance that Life offers us.

Disharmonies: *Habits that subvert or distract abilities and talents; difficulty connecting to a spiritual path; procrastination in making lifestyle changes; lethargy; procrastination in general; inability to take action due to an overactive mind and looping obsessive thoughts.*

UB-21 Stomach Connection

Virtues: This Energy Release Point empowers the integration of all forms of nourishment into all aspects of our Being. It brings us to the central core, where it connects with integrity. It serves as a physical strengthener by integrating our life experiences into a meaningful whole. It assists in keeping an impeccable alignment between our intentions, speech and actions. Unblocking and activating this Energy Release Point integrates the virtue of integrity through the virtue of being a harmonizer. By connecting to the central core, one connects to balance. From balance, the ability to rectify discrepancies between our intentions, speech and actions, by bringing us back to our centre is facilitated.

Disharmonies: *Searching for self identity; self-deprecation; self righteousness; feelings of shame; denial; to be incongruent within thought, speech and action.*

UB-22 Energy Transfer to the Three Elixir Fields

Virtues: This Energy Release Point brings balanced harmony to the full body systems empowering the virtue of love. It assists in the alignment of inner integrity of conscience, truthfulness and uprightness with communication and action. This Energy Release Point is a place of movement, bringing vitalizing transformative energy that assists in alignment to integrity. It brings clarity of connection to internal conscience so that responses in action or word manifest in congruence with one's truth. This transformative energy also empowers a strong and secure sense of individuality. This strength assists in staying in right relationship and inner fortitude to Higher Self when faced with challenging social situations as it allows for graceful flexibility in extricating oneself as the situation requires.

Disharmonies: *Weak social boundaries resulting in a compromised immune system; inability to hear one's inner voice or connect to internally generated sense of morality and conscience; deception to oneself or others.*

UB-23 Essence Palace / Tower Cover

Virtues: This Energy Release Point connects us to the palace of Life. It serves to re- energize, revitalize and balance energy from the source of raw power. It is an energy source which is abundant and accessible. Unblocking and activating this Energy Release Point re-invigorates the connection between will power and the original source of energy and purpose. It sparks the Feminine matrix of creation allowing for the flow of the Creative Force to energize the body, ignite desire and enthusiasm for life and the creative process.

Disharmonies: *Devitalization; overwhelm; fatigue; exhaustion; lethargy and procrastination; fear; stagnation which can manifest physically as kidney stones; behaviours and habits that continually lead to burnout and exhaustion.*

UB-24 Sea of Energy

Virtues: This Energy Release Point evokes the image of water, in particular the evidence of it's energy. This evidence of energy manifests at times as great agitation and waves, stormy grey and windy, or calm and sunny. Regardless of the weather, the sea carries an energy of excitement. It is vast, it is deep, it invites one to immerse in the depths and float on the foam. The sea has vast potential of life, and connecting with this Energy Release Point allows for the building and strengthening of both the feminine and masculine energies to bring forth new forms and creations in a balanced way. This is an alchemical point to help transform and re-create perspectives in life experience. Unblocking and activating this Energy Release Point connects us with the many truths of the sea. Its alchemical ability to transform and present itself in a multitude of ways, while keeping contact with its raw potential of power within its depths. With this new perspective, one can tap into and use the alchemical furnace to rebuild and restore vital life energy.

Disharmonies: *Misperceptions of reality leading to physical depletion and fatigue.*

UB-25 Large Intestine Connection

Virtues: This Energy Release Point removes blockages and obstacles which create stagnation in the flow of life. It strengthens the ability to bare life's burdens. The bowels of the body metaphorically correspond to the bowels of the Earth. The place where things are in the dark, buried and hidden from view. Connecting to this Energy Release Point assists in bringing light into the depths. It helps with the reconciliation of past behaviours and past experiences, as experiences from which one extracts the jewel of wisdom from which to learn and grow. In this perspective, one begins to understand the behaviour and aspects of being that are in the current timeframe, and in this new awareness, can bring healing light to those experiences which have caused pain in the past by embracing the shadows. It brings to conscious awareness the perception and understanding that by being responsible means to truly assess one's ability to respond in an appropriate manner. Once this perception is achieved, one can discern with wisdom and clarity what is extraneous and can finally be released, and what is essential and thereby serve as healing gems. Unblocking and activating this Energy Release Point strengthens the ability to release the extraneous in order to allow for a lightness of Being. It renews buoyancy of the body and Soul, thus empowering the ability to flow unfettered and free.

Disharmonies: *Repression of the emotional shadow leading to explosive outbursts; control issues; feelings of overwhelm which threaten to flood the full body system leading to apathy, stagnation, emptiness and loneliness; self-righteousness; martyrdom and perfectionism.*

UB-26 Primordial Gate Connection

Virtues: This Energy Release Point denotes a mysterious passageway referred to within ancient writings as a gateway between Being and Non-Being. It is a space of undifferentiated potential; a reference to the Gate of Incarnation. Gates in this context, refer to hinged barriers which can either create entrances or exits. What they open to are usually sacred spaces wherein transformation can occur. As such, Primordial Gate Connection helps regulate all other gate points in the body, so that transformative processes can occur with harmonious flow while keeping a balanced state. This Energy Release Point helps one to access the raw power of the Divine Feminine and Divine Masculine energies. Unblocking and activating this

Energy Release Point strengthens vitality drawn from a balanced source, so that it can resurrect and fuel inner strength of purpose.

Disharmonies: *Isolation; alienation from the body; fear of intimacy; withdrawal; lack of connection; anxiety; unclear sense of purpose; not living full potential.*

UB-27 Small Intestine Connection

Virtues: This Energy Release Point serves to strengthen the immune system by facilitating clear sorting processes. It is a subtle, yet clear, connection to the small intestine, whose bodily function is to separate nutrients from the whole, so that the digestive flow can continue through to elimination of the extraneous. It empowers the ability to learn what is of value and therefore discern what needs to be let go. This is a vital role in the functioning of the body, for it is through the virtues of clarity, purity and refinement that all body systems find harmony. When one can clearly distinguish what is of good in their life, and release the elements which bog down the mind and the body, the jewel of joy is more easily felt and life flows with enthusiastic purpose. Unblocking and activating this Energy Release Point allows for the full body systems to circulate with vital life force energy. An energy that has been purified and refined so that one feels an abundant flow of vitality to complete one's tasks.

Disharmonies: *Compromised immune system; seeing life as mundane; joyless; apathetic.*

UB-28 Bladder Connection

Virtues: This Energy Release Point assists with the flowing and stretching of time. It connects with the ability of immersing oneself in life, flowing through activities and yet staying fully aware of the subtleties and gentleness of the present so that the Self remains receptive to the unfolding moment. When one feels peace within, there is centre. Within centre, the ability to observe, assess and prepare for situations that arrive is strengthened. Obstacles are perceived as detours and the ability to be flexible and change directions comes with more ease. Unblocking and activating this Energy Release Point allows one to be at ease with the passage of time. It empowers the virtues of patience and calm, and strengthens the ability to be flexible in one's plans and structures so that inner peace predominates.

Disharmonies: *Internal pressure leading to anxiety; internal pressure which is out of proportion to reality and timelines; unbalanced sense of urgency; lower back pain; overwhelm and struggle to keep head above water; inability to cope with the pace of life and others.*

UB-29 Central Backbone Strength

Virtues: This Energy Release Point communicates with the strength and flexibility of the backbone. It speaks to the strength of the physical body as well as the strength of one's character. It enhances the ability to stay in centre and balance while maintaining flexibility. Strength of character is determined by the ability to be in centre, following one's integrity and inner guidance. The bones give the body structure in order to walk a path in balance. The backbone also represents the central axis of the body, and as such, contains the integrated masculine strength of endurance, fortitude and action with the feminine strength of yielding and flexibility within surrender. Unblocking and activating this Energy Release Point connects with core integrity. It assists in standing up for one's Self, one's beliefs and one's truth. It provides support for flexible feminine movement within masculine fortitude, balancing these two opposites so that a centred Self knows when to endure and persevere and when to yield and receive help.

Disharmonies: *Inflexible in body and mind; inability to take a stand for oneself; inability to "stand for something" resulting in "falling for anything"; easily swayed to the causes of others; compromise of integrity; physical mani-festation of lower back pain; compromised range of motion.*

UB-30 White Jade Ring

Virtues: This Energy Release Point refers to where the body's essence is stored. This ring encircles six powerful energies: wisdom, vital energy, willpower, soul vision, the sacred door of life, and regulates the door of release. Energies embodied by the heart, the kidneys, the spleen, the liver, the genitals and the anus. White Jade Ring empowers the strength of communication and flow between these energies with the purity of the colour white, such as found in silk, and the qualities of preciousness that are contained in the jade crystal. This Energy Release Point asks one to perceive and feel the beauty of pure white silk and jade. The softness, the strength and the richness. It becomes a metaphor for the union of opposites such as giving and receiving, masculine and feminine, soft and hard. The circuit of the six powerful energies maintains and fuels itself through the self generation of continual movement and interaction within the energies themselves. Unblocking and activating this Energy Release Point helps one to retain and hold onto what is of value in life. It strengthens the courage to see oneself in the full truth of sacredness. It is the embodiment of opposites, found within the continuous flow of integrated wholeness. It is the richness of realization of value - the beholding of oneself as a treasure, as an expression of the I AM as embodied within the sacred heart. It builds self respect, self acceptance and self love. It empowers self realization through pure devotion to the Divine. It assists in being receptive and balances this gentle receptivity with forthright action. It strengthens the stability of knowing our place in the world. Through this knowing, one builds confidence. Through confidence, healthy social interactions are supported and enthusiasm for heart filled service is strengthened.

Disharmonies: *Survival consciousness; retentive; obsessive fixation; inability to form social bonds; homelessness and dislocation; inability to connect with the wisdom of the heart; low self esteem; self deprecation; lack of desire; lack of will; lack of vision; depression; physical manifestation of anal disorders - such as cramps or painful defecation; urinary incontinence; for women - utero-vaginal inflammation; excessive uterine bleeding.*

UB-31 Upper Foramen, Upper Bone Hole / Upper Hole

Virtues: This Energy Release Point speaks to the bone where there is the sound of the wind. It represents one of the eight immortal caves through which one can access the eight original cells of creation- that is connection with The Divine Matrix. Unblocking and activating this Energy Release Point assists in harmonizing the flow of life path with the energy of knowing our purpose and destiny. This comes with a clarity and strength of purpose and by activating this reconnection, revitalization, regeneration and the ability of the body to self heal is enhanced.

Disharmonies: *Physically manifesting as lower back pain and sacrum pain, lacking motivation for wellness.*

UB-32 Second Sacral Opening

Virtues: This Energy Release Point is located on the sacrum. It is the second foramen, representing a hole or an opening to a passageway. The sacral bone has also been named the sacred bone because it holds the collected memories of genetic lineage, hence the jewels of wisdom drawn from the experience of life. In addition, the sacral bone houses the openings to the Eight Caves of Immortality. In mythology, each cave is under the protection of a Deity. Seekers of truth and wisdom would present themselves for initiation to the Mysteries of Immortality. This Energy Release Point is the second opening of initiation - the passage to wisdom. Second Sacral Opening strengthens receptivity and illumination of the personal, little mind, to open up and connect with the wisdom light of the Divine Mind. It is therefore a balanced relationship between Heaven and Earth. It is the One becoming Two in the creation of duality and the ability to remain in centre on the continuum. Second Sacral Opening also strengthens reflection of the perfect self-consciousness of the I AM Presence. Wisdom, therefore, is the mirror in which the I AM can see itself. In this aspect, it addresses two of the universal laws: the first: the Law of Attraction, which states that what is hidden within will dictate what will appear on the outside; and two: the Law of Vibration, which states that one creates or attracts the events and people who come into our life by the vibrations emitted by thoughts, words and actions. Unblocking and activating this Energy Release Point brings the seeker to understand the Mysteries through the passageway of receptive wisdom and self reflection. It brings strength to the virtues of balance. Through balance, the realization is made that there is a sense of order and a rhythmic universal breath that enables us to remain strong and flexible within the flow of life.

Disharmonies: *Inflexibility; closed mind; polarized thinking; pain in the sacrum; atrophy in the lower limbs; loss of range of motion in the lower back.*

UB-33 Centre of the Sacral Bone

Virtues: This Energy Release Point brings forward to consciousness the absolute knowing of one's sacredness. It is through this understanding that one can conceptualize the Divinity within, as well as understand that the physical body is the temple of the I AM Presence. With this awareness, the ability to understand the principle of moderation and its role in creating balance, centre and harmony within one's life experience is heightened. St. Hildegard von Bingen abbess, mystic and healer taught the principles of moderation. In her teachings, moderation is emphasized as the key to a long, healthy and joy filled life. This principle keeps life in check, to avoid extremes and to be temperate in conduct and expression. It keeps one on the path of Truth and Integrity. Unblocking and activating this Energy Release Point contributes to the ability to stand upright with strength, flexibility and balance. It upholds our alignment to our Inner Truth. Decisions and actions flow purposefully towards walking the Path with integrity, honour and self respect.

Disharmonies: *Tension causing physical pain in the sacrum; rigidity; atrophy in the lower limbs; tension; over striving; living excessively exhibiting the -aholic tendencies (for example workaholic, alcoholic, shopaholic etc)*

UB-34 Lower Sacral Bone

Virtues- This Energy Release Point is located on the sacral bone. The sacrum is viewed as the key holder of all knowledge and home to the Eight Caves of Immortality. It is the sacred bone. This Energy Release Point grounds the esoteric wisdom of the Soul into the Earth. It assures that the physical vehicle feels stable and secure. It draws on the wisdom of the Soul, and integrates our life records and experiences from our genetic lineage, so that we feel connected with humanity with compassionate understanding of the human condition. Unblocking and activating this Energy Release Point assists us to heal ourselves. It allows for reconnection to our purpose and our place within the intricate webbing/filaments of cosmic interconnections. As we heal ourselves, we heal our relationship to family. We become a whole within our individuality and then a whole within the wholeness of family. By extension, the sense of security through wholeness communicates to the betterment of community and a continual progression in evolution to the world self. At the pinnacle of expression, there is a heightened consciousness and understanding of the underlying principal of unity and the ALL is in ALL.

Disharmonies: *Physical, emotional, mental and spiritual pain; atrophy; stagnation; inability to move outside our perception and limited consciousness; alienation from others; insecurity; discomfort with others; emotional distancing.*

UB-35 Gathering of Masculine Strength and Vitality

Virtues: This Energy Release Point brings together the strength and vitality of forthright masculine energy. An energy that is sun radiant and active. An energy that is willing to partner up, co-operate and share its vitality and support when needed. It is an Energy Release Point that encourages the shifting of awareness from that of self serving Egotism of attachment to the material of the physical plane, to that of a transpersonal altruism. In this way, solar strength and forces of light generated by connection to Higher Self emanate from the Will. Vitality is drawn forth from a deep reservoir of energy and flows forward where it is needed. Unblocking and activating this Energy Release Point strengthens the will and its connection to Divine Will, effectively spiritualizing the Ego. It brings motivation, enthusiasm, endurance and determination to seize the opportunities which present and to fulfill goals.

Disharmonies: *Weakness of will; lack of motivation; expression; pain in the lower back and legs.*

UB-36 Attached Branch

Virtues: This Energy Release Point helps in the understanding and healing of family relationships and connections. Every Soul wishes to feel a sense of belonging to family: whether it be the physical family, a soul group community family, the spiritual family or world community family. This sense of belonging to a family helps establish feelings of security and stability. Feelings that are felt in a healthy childhood and contribute to the wellbeing and functioning of a strong and stable adulthood. Attached Branch strengthens healthy functioning so that problem solving is easy and puzzling events and perceived obstacles are unravelled, solved and removed. Unblocking and activating this Energy Release Point reminds us that family is found in the heart space and that we are all connected in the frequency of love. The virtue of trust in the goodness of others is restored as the energies of cooperation and community is supported.

Disharmonies: *Afflicted personal relationships; viewing people as a pain in the neck; feelings of disconnect and abandonment; not feeling one's sense of place within the family group, the community, or the larger context of the world.*

UB-37 Door of the Corporeal Soul

Virtues: This Energy Release Point connects to the force that animates the physical body. It speaks to the manifestation and vitality of the body, harmonized with the will and strength of the emotional and mental bodies.

This entity is a guardian for the body and helps to oversee inspiration, as drawn in through the lungs, and integrates inspiration with will forces so that heavenly directives can manifest. It is to be strong yet flexible, knowing and accepting limits. The importance of this Energy Release Point is it's strength in the ability to let go. When we choose to transition from the third dimensional plane, the Door of the Corporeal Soul opens and all within us which represents the mundane, exits through the anus and returns to the earth. Unblocking and activating this Energy Release Point assists in the release of what no longer serves as well as attachments. It is an Energy Release Point that assists one to let go of those who have passed on, empowering healthy grieving. It helps one to distinguish the immortality of the Soul from the temporal personality in order to contact the true spiritual ego.

Disharmonies: *Grief; inability to let go of things past; overly attached to those who have passed; fear of death; feeling spiritually empty and alone; lack of inspiration; overwork leading to depletion and de-vitalization; inner weakness.*

UB-38 Connection to the Richness of the Vital Region

Virtues: This Energy Release Point connects to the region just below the heart in the physical body. As such, it refers to various vital centres, the concept itself implying to go deep within the most fundamental regions of the body: the secret chamber of the heart where the temple of light is housed, the energetic spaces of alchemy, as well as the gateway of interface between the physical body and the etheric body. This is a very sacred Energy Release Point for it helps open the pathway, allowing for the release of Karmic stagnation. Karmic stagnation is fatalistic for it behaves as poison in the Soul. Unblocking and activating this Energy Release Point allows for a glimpse of light inside the dark aspects of the Soul, darkness which festers as poison. It brings courage to see what one is now ready to see, so that it can be revealed, explored, healed and released.

Disharmonies: *Dark secrets that fester; unexplained feelings of gloom and despair; suicidal thoughts and tendencies; deep depression; unexplained diseases.*

UB-39 Soul Hall

Virtues: This Energy Release Point anchors the realization of the sacredness of Being. From this awareness, the connection to the inner chamber of the heart is strengthened. Once this is established, the ego personality has the opportunity to exercise it's ability to make higher choices. Choices that empower and nourish the Essence of the Soul. The Soul continues it's evolution, and through the gift of Free Will, can subsequently direct focused forces for self actualization and full expression. Unblocking and activating this

Energy Release Point promotes the realization of sacredness within the self. It allows access to the passion needed for the fulfillment of purpose and destiny, stored within the inner chamber of the heart.

Disharmonies: *Disconnection from life purpose; feelings of abandonment from the spiritual world; deep melancholia.*

UB-40 Wail of Grief

Virtues: This Energy Release point empowers stability through the movement of emotions. Emotions are an integral part of the health of the inner life. The emotion of sadness is one that is felt at full intensity, however, once it begins to flow, space is created which allows other emotions to flow in their time as necessary. This Energy Release Point is also a command point for the back, helping one to stand strong and balanced, holding centre and integrity while moving through the process of releasing grief. Unblocking and activating this Energy Release Point helps provide the inner stability needed to move through intense emotions. By strengthening our stance, and staying in our centre, we become the master of these overwhelming emotions rather than the servant of them. Intense emotions can move through in a balanced way.

Disharmonies: *Overwhelmed by grief, anxiety, or fear; difficulty keeping centred; weak-kneed; self-destructive tendencies leading to loss of control. Physical manifestation of frequent urination; loss of bladder control; as well unexplained swellings.*

UB-41 Diaphragm Border

Virtues: This Energy Release Point assists in stabilizing and harmonizing movement created through the release of emotions. In this way, it is an appropriate partner to the Energy Release Point UB-40 Wail of Grief. The diaphragm is a network muscle which supports the lungs. It allows for the movement of inspiration and exhalation, providing stability and fluidity. It is a constant calming force. It serves as a pivotal transformational point so that vitality, flexible force and calming strength serve to harmonize with the lungs and heart centre, to assist in the navigation through the changes life brings. Unblocking and activating this Energy Release Point helps harmonize the movement necessary to move through transformation brought on by life experience. It allows a fluidity to the release of emotion while creating vitality and enthusiasm for the life experience.

Disharmonies: *Feelings of being stuck and un-motivated; weakness; inability to catch one's breath; inability to breath in inspiration and release the unnecessary; anxiety and fear.*

UB-42 Gate of the Ethereal Soul

Virtues: This Energy Release Point connects to the central core and vision of the inner Essence - the Soul. It is the immortal seed of the I AM Presence and encompassed within the Three Fold Flame. It is the Soul Essence which upon death of the physical, returns via Christ Consciousness to the Eternal. It connects with vision and purpose bringing guidance on the path of the incarnated lifestream. Unblocking and activating this Energy

Release Point reconnects the lifestream to vision and purpose. A vision which easily allows us to see the beauty of the world. A world in which we fully come to realize the value of our participation in what we bring to it, therefore activating the desire to create and live in the highest integrity. The realization that we are at one with humanity, and therefore, our contributions serve to benefit the whole. It penetrates to the inner recesses of the Soul to bring light, calmness, peace and joy to life. It reinforces the ability to discern and let go of what no longer serves in order to live a purposeful life.

Disharmonies: *Disconnection with purpose; feeling empty and depressed; deep sadness and longing for something more; grief; inability to let go of pre-occupation with the mundane; choosing not to evolve by clinging to the past; grief associated with the inability to let go of those who are no longer in our lives; inability to connect with the eternal truth; lack of inspiration and desire; apathy and resignation; feeling worn down by chronic illness.*

UB-43 Net of Masculine Essentials of Energy

Virtues: This Energy Release Point describes the intricate weaving of the network of life. It is a synthesizer, bringing together the plan of our life, the vision of the Soul and fluidity of energy. These three essentials synthesize to bring forth both vitality and structure in our manifestation of destiny. The synthesis of essentials is to empower the ability to make clear decisions within the process of understanding what is essential. It is precisely essential awareness that releases non-serving, illusory aspects within the personality, which allows for transformation and re-birth. Life is filled with opportunities and re-birthing moments and it is to distinguish these opportunities from the subtle influences that serve to distract along the way. Unblocking and activating this Energy Release Point provides mental clarity, objectivity, discernment and focus. It energizes forward movement and purposeful activity towards manifestation of Soul vision.

Disharmonies: *Rigidity in thought; judgmental attitude; inability to take decisive action; inability to make decisions; lack of clarity; narrow scope of vision.*

UB-44 Dwelling Place of Thought

Virtues: This Energy Release Point assists in harmonizing our thought process to be in flow with how we move through life. It allows for perception into how we extract nourishment from our life experience, so that by refining experience into purity of higher consciousness, one can create action in the world that aligns with intention. Unblocking and activating this Energy Release Point provides balance between lethargy and obsessive/compulsive behaviour so that productive action and contribution to life can ensue.

Disharmonies: *Apathy; lethargy; procrastination; inability to take action; obsessive thoughts; self-destructive tendencies; being self centred; obstinance.*

UB-45 Stomach Granary of Gold

Virtues: This Energy Release Point provides access to spiritual nourishment, the nourishment which comes from acknowledging the presence of Spirit and its life giving principle as the movement of the Soul. The Soul invites us to experience life in all its aspects, such as events, people and emotions. When one connects to Soul there is joy, purpose, security and trust. Unblocking and activating this Energy Release Point opens up the ability to receive nourishment by reconnecting to Divine Love. It allows the processing of life so that one can see the beauty and perfection of the experience. It teaches one to recognize what one needs in order to flow nourishment from within. Life becomes purposeful. The self is strengthened in unwavering trust and knowing that it is held in the secure embrace of the Divine.

Disharmonies: *Neglect of self; inability to find pleasure in a job well done; lack of compassion; callousness; needy behaviour. Physical manifestation of eating disorders and weak digestion.*

UB-46 Gate of Energy to the Vital Centres

Virtues: This Energy Release Point is a gateway to an etheric entity or interface between the physical and the non-physical, which nourishes the healthy functioning of the internal organs, in particular the area between the heart and the diaphragm. It is the passageway from the energy body which communicates information from the body elemental and the body innate to the physical body. It is the streaming energy responsible for the pulse of life found in the depths of the heart. It harmonizes the pulse of life with the rhythm of the lungs so that, through breath, we are enriched by inspiration and through pulse, we are moved to experience the wonders of life. It brings light into the density of the body. This light is a sparkling vital force that enriches the vital organs to function optimally and to circulate light through cellular structures. The circulation of light brings youthful regeneration, activates the body's ability to self heal and restores vitality. The Gate of Energy to the Vital Centres anchors light into the body as a force of illuminated consciousness. By illuminating consciousness, it becomes easier to recognize and release Karma which stagnates Soul evolution. Opening the Gate creates connection to passion and desire, and ignites creativity towards manifestation of purpose and the ultimate return to the Source. Unblocking and activating this Energy Release Point strengthens the links of communication between the etheric and physical bodies, giving the power and force necessary to embrace life with enthusiastic vitality. It enhances the ability to flow with the rhythm of life; taking in the essential for joyful nourishment and releasing that which does not serve towards living a purpose filled life. Gate of Energy to the Vital Centres brings conscious awareness and illumination through the passages of unlimited potential and possibilities via the depths of the heart.

Disharmonies: *Devitalization; psychic and physical vulnerability; fear; premature aging; feeling dull.*

UB-47 Chamber of the Will / Room of Potential

Virtues: This Energy Release Point assists in empowering clear decision making as well as activating the Will to pursue one's goals. It strengthens connection to purpose, promoting desire into meaningful action with determination in order to realize potential. Potential is inherent in all Beings. It is a reservoir of energy that when sparked, creates a momentum and expression of the Universal Principle of Action. It is Action from the certainty of Inner Knowing. Unblocking and activating this Energy Release Point strengthens the pathway connecting the mind with the heart. In this way, ultimate fulfillment of destiny through the remembrance of one's true nature and soul expression is realized and fully expressed as outward action to the world.

Disharmonies: *Hesitation; indecision; procrastination; inflexibility.*

UB-48 Vital Centre of Womb and Heart

Virtues: This Energy Release Point connects to the vitality found in the power of water - the seas in particular. It is a force of vision, passion, the rawness of where sensuality meets sexuality and through Desire births ultimate creative power. It is the same energy which conceives ideas or conceives a child. Unblocking and activating this Energy Release Point reconnects and integrates heart energies with that of the vital energy centre (the Sacral energy centre - or second energy centre). This connection and integration is necessary, for passion and desire are key elements in directing the creative forces to higher consciousness and action. This activation also incorporates the ability for a person to self nurture. This is a place of transformational energy allowing for the heart to make contact and experience emotional intimacy. By integrating the upper and lower energy centres the sexual experience becomes an intimately sacred heart connection.

Disharmonies: *Disconnection and polarization of spirituality and sexuality; traumatized sexual relationships; betrayal in intimate relationships;*

trauma of abortion or miscarriage; physical manifestation of infertility; inability to achieve orgasm; lower back pain.

UB-49 The Sequence of Orderly Boundaries

Virtues: This Energy Release Point addresses the idea of boundaries, setting a limit, having orderliness, as well as being at the end of something and on the verge of something new. This something new can be the discovery of a perspective or lifestyle resulting from the awareness that something needs to change in the way one interacts with the world. This Energy Release Point flows energy along the back and assists in flowing energy into the leg. The Energy Release Channel of the Urinary Bladder is the manifestation of the water element. Water has the ability to flood plains and fields washing away debris as well as homes and people, livestock and crops. The nature of water is to flow, however, when properly channeled in an orderly fashion, its great energy can flow to be of benefit to all parts of a landscape, encouraging fertile rich growth. Areas of excess water as well as places that are impoverished can be balanced and harmonized to bring stability in all aspects. Water also addresses connection to Source - the Ocean of Consciousness - which is interconnected with the flow of Spirit and the womb of life. By channeling this primordial energy of Source through our spiritual, mental, emotional and physical bodies, the ability to live life with ease and grace is enhanced. Circulation of the principle of reciprocity is supported in that one can ascertain and understand what is essential to one's Being. With this understanding, the ability to present and manifest our gifts and live purposefully in service to humanity and the earth will be empowered. Furthermore, there is an establishment of clarity to know how our gifts can be developed, which best benefits the needs of others. Our place in the world and how we contribute to the growth of self and others brings satisfaction and contentment. Unblocking and activating this Energy Release Point strengthens healthy boundaries so that we can be of benefit to others, through the care of self first. It creates the ability to live with fluidity and flexibility. Life becomes balanced as a result of being orderly and disciplined from within. Excesses are moderated. Rhythm is established between receiving what is essential and releasing what is inessential. Richness of the nourishing elements of water's interaction with the Earth can be more easily absorbed and the ability to stand, strongly rooted in life, flourishes.

Disharmonies: *Giving without discrimination; lack of boundaries leading to depletion and/or exhaustion; pain in the lower back; alternating constipation and diarrhea.*

UB-50 Receive Support

Virtues: This Energy Release Point provides a balanced strength by opening up the ability to receive support. It softens the naturally strong capacities of endurance and perseverance in order to balance these qualities with that of gentle surrender. It enriches the qualities of community and family by bringing the awareness that one need not bare burden alone. This burden can be in the form of physical loads as well as be in the form of emotional trauma and pain. Physically, this Energy Release Point strengthens the back by moving the energy to connect heavenly inspiration with physical vitality, to serve with expression from the heart. This facilitates the ability to live our purpose as an example of a pillar of strength. Unblocking and activating this Energy Release Point assists in the release of trauma and emotional pain, which manifests physically as pain in the back, by opening to receive the support of others. It helps one to acknowledge the needs of the emotional body, as well as honour the needs of the physical body by recognizing limits and fatigue. It empowers the ability to give oneself permission to ask for help and support, as well as honouring the process of learning to nurture oneself, in order to better be of service and a pillar of strength to others.

Disharmonies: *Emotional trauma stored deep within the muscles and bones - causing physical back pain as well as emotional pain; overwhelm.*

UB-51 Gate of Abundance

Virtues: This Energy Release Point promotes the flourishing and flowing of energy throughout the body, so that one can bring to fruition and manifestation the desires of the heart. It promotes communication between the expressions of the emotional mind such as joy, abundance and prosperity consciousness, with the passions and the desires of the heart. The name Gate of Abundance evokes the image of opening a doorway to a new level of consciousness of unlimited potential and possibility. It is a place without fear of failure, and embraces the energy of momentum and flow to step into living purposefully. It brings into perceptive awareness the recognition of the beauty and abundance that abounds all around us. When one can recognize the abundance in all things, more and more becomes visible to our awareness, creating a shift in how one approaches life. Unblocking and activating this Energy Release Point is similar to turning a key. It is a turning point, a moving into a higher level of joy. It brings motivation to embrace life with renewed interest in the world and in others. It restores the vital forces necessary to find the true meaning of love, through joy of creation and manifestation, through serving the world via the heart.

Disharmonies: *Resignation and apathy; depression and despair; poverty consciousness; lack of connection to desire and emotion in order to fuel the passion of the heart; physical manifestation of sciatica.*

UB-52 Floating Reserves of Energy

Virtues: This Energy Release Point addresses the ability to float upon the current of life. The current of life is likened to streams, lakes and waterways which can be at times tranquil or very dynamic. Regardless of the water surface, great currents of energy abound within its depths. To float on this current, one must be able to remain light and buoyant. This Energy Release Point helps one to sustain joy within the heart by the infusion of buoyancy, courage and optimism. It strengthens the ability to remain in the present moment, flowing with life and navigating changes as they come. It assists with remaining balanced, calm, and heart centred.

Unblocking and activating this Energy Release Point helps one to observe the changes around them, within a space of contemplation and joyful buoyancy. It assists with connecting to the deeper wisdom of the Heart, and replenishing oneself with the reserves of energy found within the depths of streaming currents, so that one can navigate the circumstances which greet us along life's journey.

Disharmonies: *Inflammation in the rear of the knee; inflexibility; lack of movement; heavy heartedness; discouragement; emotional attachments; longing for the past.*

UB-53 Balance of Masculine Energy

Virtues: This Energy Release Point is a harmonizer that serves to restore the balance of energy. It is a meeting place of where two opposites collide and create chaos. The image one senses when connecting to this Energy Release Point is that of water, represented by the Energy Release Channel of the Urinary Bladder, and that of fire, represented by the Energy Release Channel of the Three Elixir Fields. As a harmonizer, it accesses quiet still-ness found in the centre of the chaos so that preparations for what is to come can be formulated with clear intention as connected to purpose. It is within stillness that one can observe the dynamics of change. It is within stillness that one can connect to the impulses which serve to spark vital forces of movement. In this way, intention and clarity of purpose is fuelled with energy that supports our mission when we step into life. Unblocking and activating this Energy Release point provides access to inner stillness so that one can consciously formulate intentions, all while being able to access the dynamic energy needed to manifest action.

Disharmonies: *Fear; inability to stay calm and centred during times of stress; feelings of overwhelm during multi-levelled activity; feeling tension and pain in the lower back; pain and stiffness in the lower limbs; inflamma-tion of the kidneys.*

UB-54 Central Equilibrium

Virtues: This Energy Release Point connects to the strength of centre within our core and furthers this strength by empowering our core connection with the core of the Earth. The Earth element is one of stability and foundation. Central Equilibrium allows us to face fear, quell worry and balance overwhelm from a centre of stability. In this place of stability we take decisive action and delegate priorities to the proper spheres of action. Unblocking and activating this Energy Release Point allows us to use the energy of fear to teach us what we need to address and conquer. In so doing, we move forward in our evolution towards mastery with equilibrium and centre.

Disharmonies: *Frustration; feeling like we are drowning; anxiety; easily overwhelmed; feeling over extended; inappropriate boundaries; feelings of fragility. Physical manifestation of loss of bladder control.*

UB-55 Unified Forces

Virtues: This Energy Release Point brings together the culmination of strength and power of the forward thrust of masculine energy within the Creative Force. It is an energy of strength within fluidity and movement. It is an energy which strengthens and supports the activities of life, filling them with Sun Source Vitality. Unblocking and activating this Energy Release Point empowers the energy of active strength found within the physical body, and actively integrates and unifies this strength within the full body systems. Once this energy circulates through, this Energy Release Point directs energy to ground Spirit into the physical earth. Unified Forces solidifies the ability to stand strong in the remembrance that each individual is an embodiment of the I AM spark of creation. It enhances the connection to the foundational support of the Creative Force for the active manifestation of our potential in the world.

Disharmonies: *Inability to move forward in purposeful action; feeling unsupported; generalized weakness of the legs; inability to feel grounded.*

UB-56 Supporting Muscles

Virtues: This Energy Release Point serves to support the muscles of the legs so that in turn, the legs support us in carrying our gifts of service into the world. It builds inner strength to support the physical, so that one feels productive and motivated to continue. This Energy Release Point has a continual effect, for by strengthening the muscles, the perseverance and discipline of the mind is also affected. A secondary aspect of this Energy Release Point is that by connecting to the discipline of the mind, the light within the mind connects to the point of light within the Universal Divine Mind. This allows for an opening that receives Light strength, a strength which affirms the knowing that one is always supported by the Divine. When we have clear connection that our acts of productivity are in alignment with Divine Will, then the resulting manifestation will be fuelled from benevolence for the betterment of humanity. Unblocking and activating this Energy Release Point strengthens the will to be of service, and supplies the vital support necessary to the physical structure so that it can step into benevolent action.

It allows for balanced communication between the mind and the needs of the physical body so that both are respected and honoured.

Disharmonies: *Imbalanced support for the body by constant mind over matter leading to depletion and exhaustion of the physical as well as exhaustion of the mental; disorders of digestion and the intestines.*

UB-57 Supporting Mountain

Virtues: This Energy Release Point is the strength of the mountain. It is endurance and perseverance. It is mental sharpness and discernment. It signifies the ability of enormous achievement. It is likened to a pillar of strength that is capable of holding together a body, a family and a community by providing structure, stability and balance. Unblocking and activating this Energy Release Point strengthens one's core with firmness of integrity, and through discernment, allows for the release of what is extraneous. This release is necessary in order for one to flow in a strong, integral, capable manner. This pillar is then, by extension, capable of shifting in a positive manner all those around - the family, friends and by extension, the community and the world. Creation of the example of support, structure of strength, stability and balance.

Disharmonies: *Overwhelm; exhaustion; over-striving; out of balance; rigidity; unbalanced expectation of oneself or of others.*

UB-58 Take Flight and Scatter

Virtues: This Energy Release Point strengthens internally generated behaviour that modulates our ability to have a calm and steady presence in the face of fear and uncontrollable agitation. This is of vital importance in the modern day age of technology where conditions of mass consciousness thought forms disseminate with increasing rapidity serving to fuel conditions such as mass hysteria. It is said that the energy of chaos and confusion is designed to sever our connection to our Essence and ultimately the Divine. The result of this severance being uncontrolled agitation, confusion of will and intention as well as compromise in the ability to reflect and think for oneself. This Energy Release Point then serves to re-establish the connection to the Divine spark within, empowering inner calm and steady presence. It is to be inspired and realize that one may trust in a positive expectation of good will, as well as have faith in a benevolent outcome. This steadfast trust and faith grow in resonance from within and serves to radiate loving compassion and a calm presence, thereby creating an environment which serves to calm and stabilize others. This amplifies the ability to bring harmony within one's self and others in the environment. Unblocking and activating this Energy Release Point assists us in holding our vibration and resonance to light filled forces. Forces which are powerful beyond measure and bring vitality and strength to appropriate behaviour as circumstances require. It anchors the light of compassion, calm and harmony within our whole body systems. Our very presence radiates a loving, calm, compassionate self, a self which exudes peace and harmony.

Disharmonies: *To be carried away in uncontrollable agitation; fear; inability to focus; inability to find calm and centre within; anxiety; easily vulnerable to thought forms which promote chaos and fear; fainting.*

UB-59 To Access Masculine Energy

Virtues: This Energy Release Point speaks to the ability of accessing strong, forthright movement and action. Energy that is strongly associated with masculine power. Unblocking and activating this energy Release Point creates the movement to stir up, expose and release stagnation due to toxicity. This is likened to a strong light which serves to find and expose that which is hidden, bring it to awareness in order for it to be removed. To Access Masculine Energy assists in maintaining flowing active energy which serves to keep clear and remove environmental, emotional, mental and spiritual toxicity.

Disharmonies: *Attachment to co-dependent relationships; environmental sensitivity; enmeshed in a lifestyle of toxicity; congestion and inflammation in the body; stagnation.*

UB-60 Kunlun Mountain

Virtues: This Energy Release Point helps balance the way one expresses the passions of the heart. It conveys the idea of self-reflection and illumination. It promotes insight into the depths which serve to balance the receptive state of feminine awareness with forthright masculine action. It strengthens the ability to practice moderation so that there is grounded idealism. It stimulates creativity and the re-birthing process. The name Kunlun Mountain makes reference to Chinese mythology. In this myth, there are great floods of destruction and humanity is lost. The peak of Kunlun Mountain is the highest peak and the first to present as the flood waters recede. It is on this peak that the brother and sister gods of creation land. It is here that they copulate and re-kindle life with the creation of humanity. Many cultures have mythology regarding the floods, the ending of one humanity and the creation of a new humanity to repopulate the earth. The mountain becomes the symbol of wisdom, new beginnings and connection to the God-force. Kunlun Mountain is paradise. To climb Kunlun Mountain is to assure immortality as it re-unites the Cosmic Fires of Creation (found in Heaven) with the Primordial forces of water (found on earth). This is the reconnection to the seed and subsequent flowering of life. It is re-birth and resurrection. Kunlun Mountain becomes the metaphor for Ascension. Unblocking and activating this Energy Release Point activates the desire and passion to re-birth and make oneself new. It balances fear by transforming it into wisdom. It supports the process of creation and ascension, by drawing on the alchemical elements of the basis for life - feminine water integrated with the passionate fire of the masculine.

Disharmonies: *Fanaticism; resistance to change; over intensity; self righteousness; manipulative behaviour; fear; agitated nervous system; anxiety; dream disturbed sleep; cold heartedness; inability to catalyze will forces through the heart; inability to express; feelings of spiritual abandonment; inability to birth new ideas; stifled creativity.*

UB- 61 Servant's Aid / Quieting of Evil

Virtues: This Energy Release Point is the seventh point from the extremity of the Energy Release Channel of the Urinary Bladder. It is also, numerically, a number seven as it is the sixty first Energy Release Point of the Urinary Bladder. (6 + 1) The number seven is symbolic of pushing us to the next higher level of consciousness/awareness, a number of going boldly forward in the exploration of the unknown. The number seven is composed of two lines. The first line is horizontal. It represents stability and support as well as a view of the unlimited horizon. The potential of all that there is ahead of us in the journey waiting for exploration. The second line is diagonal, representing the freedom of limitation and the courage to follow one's unique path and destiny. The diagonal coming from the stability of the horizontal allows for a clear directed vision of the path. It is a deliberately drawn and manifested creation of direction. Unblocking and activating this Energy Release Point gives the strength to continue onto our destination. It is the strength of a faithful servant, one who nourishes and supports the ability to stay on the path, bringing the strength of unwavering conviction of the inner being of the lifestream so that one can express and live purposefully. Within this strength of the journey, there is an understanding, a commitment to oneself and the Divine which reassures safety, trust and success. It is the unfoldment of a perfect Lifepower, where one knows that the logical consequence of the unfoldment of ideas and plans will triumphantly manifest as they are meant to. The idea and the plan in itself is a perfect creation. As the name Quieting of Evil suggests, it releases the influences and limitations imposed by errant thought forms that torment the mind and distract one from connecting to authenticity and the vision of the Soul. It dispels enchantments, illusions and spells that cause great fear.

Disharmonies: *Undertakings that frequently fail in their final steps before completion- due to fear; attracting thought forms which perpetuate fear; easily influenced by others, thereby losing connection with authenticity and inner truth; entity invasion/possession.*

UB-62 Extended Vessel / Ghost Road

Virtues: This Energy Release Point assists in creating the space and containment required to receive, store and circulate higher wisdom and knowledge. It helps with discernment to see what is truth and how this truth is reflected in our life. To discern how we can weed out non-beneficial influences, release extraneous non-serving distractions and to retain the jewel of what is essential to the unfoldment of our life plan. The ability to receive and access Universal Truths and to consciously understand them becomes the blueprint and basis for beneficial co-creative action. Extended Vessel provides a container of resources so that we create a fulfilling life in which we not only develop our wisdom, but also transform our wisdom and Universal Truths through the extension of ourselves into the world by our acts of service to others. Unblocking and activating this Energy Release Point empowers receptivity and allows these wisdoms to flow into us and be held within stores of containment for use towards manifestation of an empowered life. In this way, we are facilitated to become conscious directors of life as well as express ourselves in service to others. As the name Ghost Road suggests, this Energy Release Point is a ghost point. It serves to release negative energies that disconnect one from inner truth, willpower and the directives of the Soul as well as blocking the ability to pay attention to the needs of the body.

Disharmonies: *Fatigue; depression; inflexibility; rigidity in the body; over-striving; inability to access clear focused thoughts. Physical manifestations of pain in the shoulders from over pushing and over work.*

UB-63 Golden Gate / Bridge Pass

Virtues: This Energy Release Point brings one to the place of ultimate safety. When one feels safe, there is security, calmness and peace. These conditions are necessary in order to receive the subtle messages of the Soul, messages which will assist in promoting a balanced flow in all aspects of life. A bridge is a structure which provides a connection between two different things. On the physical level, there are examples of bridges connecting two opposites sides of a river. In this function of connection, the bridge provides safe passage. There are, however, many aspects to a bridge. On the emotional/mental level, a bridge provides support through times of distress so that the state of calm can be restored. On the spiritual level, the bridge provides the state of ease and grace, protection and guidance during threshold experiences. It is connection with the golden light of Christ Consciousness. Golden Gate is a reference to mythology, where there is a mysterious queen mother of the West in the land of the setting sun. She is pictured as a golden gate that welcomes the souls of those who are entering the stage of completion of their life journey on the physical plane. She is beautiful, calm and loving. She baths them with her golden life giving waters so that the souls are refreshed and renewed for the next stage of their journey - re-birth into the spirit world. Unblocking and activating this Energy Release Point opens the sensory orifices for better reception of Divine messages. It promotes the ability to feel the guidance and protection of the spiritual world so that one feels ultimate safety and trust in the unfoldment of life. Perception and awareness is enhanced. Access to the flow of life giving waters brings regeneration and rejuvenation of energy, so that the ability to align with the universal rhythm of life expresses with ease and grace.

Disharmonies: *Stagnation caused by fear of the unknown; inability to embrace life due to fear; anxiety; agitated mind; overwhelm; feeling of drowning in responsibilities and life circumstances; spiritual orphan; feeling cut off from guidance; fear of death.*

UB-64 Capital Bone / Central Bone

Virtues: This Energy Release Point strengthens the circulation of energy throughout the full body systems allowing one to more clearly harmonize all the Energy Release Channels to flow with more freedom and less constraint. This creates optimum clarity, function, health and wellness within the physical, emotional, mental and spiritual bodies. Unblocking and activating this Energy Release Point further allows one to reach the very marrow of the bones, a connection which empowers security in the absolute core of one's being. This realization produces an outflow of strength, creativity and flexibility to adapt and respond to life, knowing that resources and reserves are available and constantly created. The connection to the bones serve as a reminder of our vital structure which provides protection and a framework for our journey.

Disharmonies: *Lack of structure; weakness; inflexibility; lack of clarity; dryness.*

UB-65 Bone Binder / Thorn Bone

Virtues: This Energy Release Point penetrates the depths of vision. It allows for clear connection to the source of light found deep within our bones, anchoring this light deep into the earth. Bone Binder speaks of the ability of energy to manifest and activate a cohesive entity (the Innate) to synthesize disparate elements into a living wholeness. The name Thorn

Bone extends the imagery to that of a plant that photosynthesizes light into life force energy. An energy which has major beneficial effects for the environment as well as serving to circulate essential energy throughout the plant. The plant can therefore draw strength by anchoring its roots into the depths of the earth and show its potential. Unblocking and activating this Energy Release Point removes the veils that shroud insights to the understanding of our Essence. It allows for a flowering of potential, by stimulating the growth of active intelligence - a waking consciousness. Clear vision of potential, decisiveness and inner resolve is empowered, thereby strengthening the ability to create conscious action with awareness as aligned with inner wisdom.

Disharmonies: *Constant anxiety; fear; compulsive actions which contradict our inner virtues; excessive bone growth manifesting as calcium deposits and kidney stones; spinal sterosis; heel spurs.*

UB - 66 Penetrating Valley

Virtues: This Energy Release Point quiets the nervous system so that spiritual sensitivity is enhanced. It allows for the flow of spirit to move into the valley, nourish the treasures and transform the shadows. Serenity becomes the natural state of being. It calms and soothes the mind so that one can moderate and flow energy in a graceful and balanced way. It helps one to become more aware of subtleties of spirit, helping to penetrate the shadows in the valley so that the emotional life is softened, harmonized and integrated for balanced function in life. Unblocking and activating this Energy Release Point allows light to penetrate into the valley of shadows. Sensitivity and receptivity to spiritual awareness of the gift of experience serves to strengthen the ability to heal traumas that define one's emotional history so that the shadow can be resolved, integrated or released. The focus of the will is strengthened and challenges are met directly and easily, thereby allowing the mind to be at peace.

Disharmonies: *Generalized fear and anxiety; generally high-strung; easily wound-up; inappropriate assertion of power over everything and everyone as an attempt to overcome insecurity.*

UB - 67 Extremity of the Divine Feminine Matrix

Virtues: This Energy Release Point draws energy through the womb of the Divine Feminine Matrix so that we can connect to the preciousness of our sacredness. It empowers self worth, self esteem and self confidence to connect to our full potential in order to self realize and attain the ultimate goal. It is the pivotal point of transformation of the Divine Feminine energy into the Divine Masculine energy, thereby facilitating inward movement into the depths of one's being, simultaneously empowering the outward movement necessary for transformation. It is re-birth on many levels, as it has the ability to create a powerful movement energy that serves to knock one back onto the path of Destiny, should one veer off course. It is a course corrector. In fact, the physical stimulation of this Energy Release Point has the ability on a pregnant woman (the feminine in full flower) to turn a wrongly positioned baby and facilitate labour. Unblocking and activating this Energy Release Point activates a movement energy that brings to realization that something must change. It is an active energy that prompts the removal of the veil of self deprecation and hesitation, so that one connects to their inner divinity and realizes one's sacredness and potential. It releases fear that is associated with change so that one is impelled to reach and move through the point of no return. Once achieved, there is no going back. Life moves forward, embracing the now moment with enthusiasm of what the unknown future will bring. It activates the pure raw power of the feminine creative matrix, so that one can reach the summit of perfection and culmination of self realization.

Disharmonies: *Overwhelm; caught in a cycle of patterns of abuse; lack of clarity; attachment to busy-ness as a way of escaping.*

Portraits of the Energy Release Points for the Energy Release Channel of the Kidney

KID-1 Bubbling Spring / Burst of Vibrancy

Virtues: This Energy Release Point speaks to our connection with the Great Source or Essence from which all life springs. The Source which on Earth is seen as water - life giving, purifying, vibrant and essential to our existence. We are made up of water. As water bubbles out of the ground in the form of springs, we witness the strength and vitality that is required for it to burst through layers of earth, rock and stone all the while emitting joyful music through it's bubbling sound. Many of these springs world wide have become sacred places known for miraculous and spontaneous healing. These springs are witness to the vitality and life giving healing properties made manifest from water's journey of purification through the Earth's crust and it's countless gem and mineral qualities. This Energy Release Point opens us up to the bursting energy of water's vibrancy and purity. Through unblocking and activating this Energy Release Point, we can draw into our body the vitality of Source. Our whole body systems are then refreshed and rejuvenated by the replenishment of our inner waters as the memory of water reconnects to it's origin. Through this reconnection we are inspired to receive and be infused with renewed vision and growth. We reconnect with our creativity and are propelled toward forward flow in self empowerment, grounded balance, joy and vitality, embracing higher evolution.

Disharmonies: *Lack of motivation; lack of vitality; feeling of stagnation; anxiety; depletion; disconnection from purpose; overly influenced by others.*

KID-2 Blazing Valley / Dragon in the Abyss

Virtues: This Energy Release Point evokes the image of fires blazing in a valley. Valleys are usually seen as places of lush green growth and coolness, often within the shadow of the mountains. This Energy Release Point is blazing, it is as though the dragon within the abyss has been poked or jabbed awake from it's slumber and it now rises upwards, breathing it's fire, making his presence known. Unblocking and activating this Energy Release Point unleashes the fire of the dragon. It is highly creative, transformational, magical energy with the ability to harmonize the heart with its flaming passion with wisdom as embodied by water - the source of the lush valley and the womb of the Divine Feminine. Alchemically, the dragon draws spiritual potency from these seeming opposites. In Ancient texts such as the Wang Fu in China (c.76-163 BC) it is written: Dragon fire and human fire are opposite. If dragon fire comes into contact with wetness it flames; and if it meets water it burns. If one drives it away by means of fire, it stops burning and it's flames are extinguished. Blazing Valley/Dragon in the Abyss is therefore the vision of seeing a dragon emerge from a primal whirlpool in full magnificence and strength. It is the foundation of health and immunity. It empowers illumination into our depths and redirects our consciousness to innate purpose and drive to fulfill destiny.

Disharmonies: *Introversion; depletion; exhaustion from over-striving.*

KID-3 Great Mountain Stream

Virtues: This Energy Release point is the source of all Energy. It connects one to the great Universal ALL - the Creative Force from which all things come. This Great Mountain Stream has the ability to nourish and vitalize all the streams, rivers and lakes that stem from it. Despite this torrential power it is a balanced source of strength, promoting stillness as well as a quiet meditative mind. Unblocking and activating this Energy Release Point connects us to the vitality and nourishment of this active living water. Streaming down from the top of the mountain, gathering force in its journey to connect life force with our physicality. When centre and stillness is found, fear is released and wisdom of the Heart can be heard. Vitality is renewed in order to fulfill destiny.

Disharmonies: *Overwhelming fear; inability to recognize and grow our gifts; wasting our potential; neediness and worry promoting fear.*

KID-4 Great Bell

Virtues: The function of a bell is to call. It is to summon all souls to an event. This could be a communal gathering to discuss social or political events or a celebratory festive occasion. The Great Bell signifies the Call to something that is even more extraordinary - a transformational spiritual movement towards a calling to purpose that is of such magnitude that one cannot ignore or refuse. This Energy Release Point moves all obstacles which block the expression of inborn potential. It is a gate within the depths of the Soul that when opened clears away all negative influences that obscure our awareness and insight into our original Essence. When the Great Bell is ignored, when one resists or struggles against the current of movement to SOUL - this bell becomes an Alarm Bell - a portent of oncoming distress which can manifest as a physical imbalances leading to a life threatening illness. Hence the expression "For Whom the Bell Tolls" - John Donne (1572-1631), the first of metaphysical poets.

"Perchance be for whom this bell tolls may be so ill, as that he knows not it tolls for him; and perchance I may think myself so much better than I am, as that they who are about me, and see my state, may have caused it to toll for me, and I know not that."

The revelation being that serious illness can bring metamorphic transformational change. Unblocking and activating this Energy Release Point brings a calling. A calling of such power that it demands the ego to listen to the SOUL. In this way, Great Bell reconnects us to our deeper purpose and fulfillment of destiny.

Disharmonies: *Not being willing to see the reality around us; fear; struggle for survival; workaholic tendencies - to build and collect material possessions that on the physical, emotional and mental level lead to depletion as we struggle to keep our heads above water.*

KID-5 Water Spring

Virtues: This Energy Release Point unleashes the power of water in all of its forms. Water in the form of an ocean has the qualities of vastness and depth; rapids in the river has dancing vibrancy; a lake has stillness and tranquility; the fog and mist contain cloudy mysteriousness. It is the force and strength of water's purity which serve to empower and revitalize the flow of life. Unblocking and activating this Energy Release Point allows for the tapping into the reservoir of Water Spring and empowers the regeneration of body systems, bringing fluidity and flexibility in all aspects of being. In addition, the forms of water and it's qualities enhance perseverance and strength of Will. The strength of Will allows for a greater ability to break through the illusion of imprisonment and therefore empowers one's ability to manifest in all aspects of expression. Water Spring supports the flow of potential into the world.

Disharmonies: *Lack of will; devitalization; inability to move forward towards goals; inability to flow with life. Physical manifestation of pain below the heart region; difficult urination; menstrual issues.*

KID-6 Sea of Reflection and Illumination

Virtues: This Energy Release Point connects to the depths of the vast ocean of consciousness, the womb of creation, where the Divine Feminine births and generates the potentialities of the Soul. The sea is the Microcosm to the ocean and the individual is the Microcosm to the sea. The individual, therefore, is made of consciousness - as generated by the Divine Feminine and made active by the Divine Masculine. The oceans, seas, and water systems move and flow by this dynamic energy. The water itself is a reflection of both aspects of the Creative Force - for it holds depth and moisture of primordial being-ness and yet reflects light and activity of the sun, the moon and the stars as active expression of doing-ness. It is inner vitality of inner wisdom. Unblocking and activating this Energy Release Point creates the opportunity to witness the reflection of Soul self brilliance. A brilliance fuelled by illumination and wisdom. By connecting to this brilliance, the mind is illuminated to the unknown nature of Self, in all aspects - the gifts, the beauty, the fears; all that which is buried. It enables conscious connection, allowing reflection into wisdom and thereby healing and releasing that which hinders the full growth into a Self Realized Being.

Disharmonies: *Fear stemming from Karmic sources; shock; trauma; anxiety; feelings of urgency; easily overwhelmed by life circumstances.*

KID-7 Returning and Repeating Current / Beyond Destiny

Virtues: This Energy Release Point speaks to the flow of life. In physicality, there is the moment of conception, birth and death. Death on the physical plane is the point of birth in the spiritual plane and from here there is the continuation of life, to the point of descent into the physical for a returning cycle of conception, birth and re-birth. Within the cycle of life itself on the physical plane, this Energy Release Point is the place of the unification of the Divine Masculine Energy with the Divine Feminine Energy and as such rules the moment of conception. It is ultimate creative power and ultimate vitality. It is evolution and transformation powered by the creative matrix where the sperm penetrates the egg and begins the cycle of life. Unblocking and activating this Energy Release Point unleashes the potential energy, alchemically transforming it into active power that multiplies and amplifies exponentially. The alternate name, Beyond Destiny, indicates that one has come to a point of non-growth, of no return. This state having grown by blocking destiny by stagnating with living in the past, holding on to illusion, full of remorse with the missed opportunities life experience has presented. To the point that a physical illness has a life of it's own and overtakes the ability to live a purpose filled life. In this case, unblocking and activating this Energy Release Point can assist with the transition from life to death, where the cycle of the return can be re-set and re-harmonized to the re-birthing cycle.

Disharmonies: *Pre-occupation with the mundane; apathy; resignation; exhaustion leading to dis-ease; attachments to the past; inability to learn from life experiences.*

KID-8 Sincerity and Trust

Virtues: This Energy Release Point creates the pathway of connection to truth, sincerity and trust. It helps build faith and inner wisdom within self and empowers the ability to trust that communication and exchanges with others will be met with an equal measure of sincerity and truth. This Energy Release Point creates the environment for harmonious exchange where wisdom prevails and the building of security, commitment, strength, integrity, confidence, sincerity and trust flourishes. Unblocking and activating this Energy Release Point brings peace and harmony to dissolve the fear which hinders the ability to trust in the communication of our truths and to have confidence that these truths will be well received by those around us. It empowers commitment to manifest our purpose in life as communicated by heaven at the point of our conception, as well as strengthening faith in the outcomes.

Disharmonies: *Fear; anxiety; lack of confidence; expecting the worst in people and in situations; mistrust of others; betrayal issues.*

KID-9 Building Guest

Virtues: This Energy Release Point strengthens the creativity centre, creating the room for welcoming and housing a baby or for the gestation of a project, or artistic creation. This Energy Release Point empowers the continual flow of life as it takes a seed, gestates it, transforming it for birth. It is a spiritual embryo as well, incubating and awakening us to life and the pursuit of the development of our talents and cultivation of our potential, the birthing of our new self. Unblocking and activating this Energy Release Point begins the process of creating and re-birthing. One cannot conceive solely on one's own. There must be a joining of masculine and feminine energies. Likewise inspiration is received from the exterior and drawn in. The Divine Energy or breath of Spirit brings forward the awakening of creativity and flowering of potential.

Disharmonies: *Infertility on one or more levels of Being: the physical, emotional, mental and spiritual planes. Feeling unsupported; unloved; feeling of lack.*

KID-10 Valley of the Divine Feminine

Virtues: This Energy Release Point facilitates the flow of life's purpose into the world. Valley of the Divine Feminine brings strength and allows for inner illumination into the depths of one's being. From this place one can find, retrieve, and bring forward our talents and gifts. From here, one can gracefully step into the unfoldment of destiny. Unblocking and activating this Energy Release Point is likened to the powerful energy of birthing and yet done in a way of balanced gentleness and strength. The ancient precept holds true: *"Nothing under Heaven is softer or weaker than water, yet nothing can compare with it in attacking the hard and strong"* (I-Ching). This Energy Release Point serves to empower fluidity in all aspects of our Being. We are made mostly of water and our energy as connected to our physicality should flow fluidly - free of resistance and yet with steady strength - similar to a mighty river. The physical location of this point on the human body is in the crevice of the knee - mimicking nature in it's similarity to where we see a bend in the river. The river and nature know that it's path is to be at one with the ocean. The human path is also to be at One, and as we walk through the Valley of the Divine Feminine, we are given the gift of flow which assists us to move gracefully in manifestation of our purpose in life.

Disharmonies: *Overuse of will forces which are not in alignment with Divine Will; mind over-riding the needs of the body; fear and anxiety causing overwork or struggle - creating patterns of stagnation; patterns of stagnation which lead to the manifestation of feeling as though one is living in a shadow - through the life of another, or simply living a dimmed version of our potential; darkness; self created Hell which one cannot seem to escape; to be in a dilemma, a predicament or a difficult situation with the inability of seeing light in this valley of the shadows.*

KID-11 Horizontal Bone / Curved Valley

Virtues: This Energy Release Point connects to the deepest recesses of our Essence through the marrow of our bones; a place where we will never be shaken or thrown off for it is the absolute core of who we are. In reaching this place, we can cleanse and transform ourselves through the vitality likened to that of a seed bursting into life holding the inherited pattern of our potential. Here is the inner core of strength, which serves to hold our integrity while protecting our Essence. This Energy Release Point also assists with the integration of our spirituality with our physical sexual function honouring the sacred wholeness. Through conscious unity, the sexual act becomes sacred. The conception and incubation of life is likewise a sacred service of Divine love. Unblocking and activating this Energy Release point allows for the reception of Divine inspiration, enhancing the ability to bring all creative projects to fruition.

Disharmonies: *Inner torment and Hell; self destructive tendencies; suicidal thoughts; self mutilation; feelings of oppression; being enmeshed in situations of dilemma and predicaments; shame and fear associated with sexuality and sexually transmitted diseases; feelings of impotence; lack of creativity; feelings of aloneness and experiencing the valley of the shadows; feeling that life keeps throwing curves and twists on the path; polarization of sexuality and spirituality; sexual addictions.*

KID-12 Great Glorious Brightness

Virtues: This Energy Release Point empowers conception - the conception of ideas or the conception of a child. It stimulates the sexual energy centre, also known as the creativity centre, to enhance creativity and empower growth. It is the sun and it's glorious bright solar energy that, with it's warmth, allows for the growth and flowering of plants. It is also the full engagement of feminine earth energies with the masculine solar power that create the ideal environment for life and growth to flourish. Likewise, in our intimate sexual relationships, full engagement of the sexual energies in the body with that of spiritualized energy of the Divine

Masculine and Feminine forces will lead to glorious fulfillment and bliss of a sacred union. Unblocking and activating this Energy Release Point allows the solar aspects of healthy ego strength to illuminate the feminine depths within, promoting our ability to transcend fear and shame. It is the balanced ego strength that allows the transformation of fear into wisdom of the Heart. When this transformation happens, the heart unwraps itself to open, receive and share it's depths of love and authenticity with positive vulnerability. Introspection and healing warmth are activated as the heart opens to the warmth of trust. Thus commences the process of a compassionate cleansing of the subconscious of the shadow, along with integrating spirituality with sexuality.

Disharmonies: *Fear of intimacy; fear of the unknown; excessive blushing; shyness; lack of confidence; shame in regards to sexuality; coldness and frigidity; inability to relax; problems with conception.*

KID-13 Door of Infants

Virtues: This Energy Release Point opens, nourishes and encourages vital bursting of energy. It is this energy that is present and shows strength in the birthing of a baby, the blossoming of a flower and in the hatching of an egg. It is an energy that carries with it enthusiasm and curiosity embedded on the matrix of creativity. It is through this Energy Release Point that full expression of Free Will, the birthright of our individuality, manifests. Unblocking and activating this Energy Release Point strengthens vitality and initiative to burst forth and explore life with the natural freedom and curiosity of a child and thereby living a purposeful life. It furthermore assists in releasing childhood trauma, allowing for movement through fear, in order to continue and flow the path of destiny.

Disharmonies: *Fear; anxiety; exhaustion and fatigue; overly serious tendencies; workaholic tendencies; inability to play; lack of spontaneity.*

KID-14 Fullness of Four

Virtues: This Energy Release Point brings together two very important concepts; the number four as well as fullness brought by abundance and plenty. The number four represents movement. In music, intervals of the fourth were used in sacred music of the church inspiring devotion to God and connection through the gift of the Holy Spirit. Humanity has four limbs to move forward, embrace, give and receive the joys that a purposeful life brings. Movement here implies being moved by the joy of Spirit to embrace doing, living and being through our physical vehicle. Four can also be the number for balance, harmony and bringing practicality to our spiritual visions. Nature also provides the number four with producing the winds of the four directions. The winds of change create movement from the four directions and resonantly, nature transforms itself cyclically through the movement of time through the four seasons. In this cyclical movement, humanity is in the centre of the experience. The ability to navigate the movement and changes of life from a state of centre is directly related to one's inner sense of abundance and plenty, as well as being inclusive and generous of nature within grounded practicality. Unblocking and activating this Energy Release Point connects one to centre and balance, allowing the opportunity to penetrate to the inside of our Essence, nourish and fuel vitality, in order to continue forward motion in the fulfillment of desires from a place of abundance.

Disharmonies: *Fear of change; inability to flow with life; fear of lack; miserly or hoarding tendencies; stagnation; inability to serve and give to others. Physical manifestations of bloating; abdominal fullness and distention, gynaecological disorders; fibroids and barrenness.*

KID-15 Central Flow

Virtues: This Energy Release Point expresses the Esoteric Principle of the One, the point where the creative life force energy moves from the One into the becoming of the Two. The point of becoming both Masculine and Feminine as expressed by the Hidden Principle - All is gender, as well as the fourth Universal Principle of Polarity. It is to be in the centre, or in the middle, between within these Principles. Centre and middle is being in truth, in alignment, the expression of moderation, balance and harmony. It is to also have clear boundaries for empowerment of healthy, purposeful action. These are all qualities that assist in the defining of who we are and what we do. It can be expressed metaphorically as the point where life begins, it's strength derived from the ability to connect with the inherited vitality of our genetics. At this Energy Release Point one connects with the Energy Release Channel of the Penetrating Interface, a source of great vitality for creation. Unblocking this Energy Release Point brings connection with the pattern or blueprint for our life unfoldment. Activating this Energy Release Point dynamically energizes its vitality and begins the flow to action. It is truly to be a Master of Flow and Manifestation. To actively co-create with the quality of the flow of water, connect the Three Treasures of Heaven, Humanity and Earth, within all levels of our embodiment in the physical. Unblocking and activating this Energy Release Point strengthens our inner resolve, our centre. It provides the environment for participating in life through a balanced state, dissipating emotions such as fear and cleansing discordant thoughts, releasing through the quality of the flow of water that which can no longer exist when in a One-ness consciousness state. It strengthens perseverance to reach goals in a manner which is flexible and flowing harmoniously with self, with time and with others.

Disharmonies: *Extreme polarization/duality; fear; inability to move forward; inability to create; obsessive compulsive thoughts and actions; lack of compassion. Physical manifestation of painful menstrual conditions; irregular menses; lower abdominal pain; constipation; inflammation and swelling of joints; sore lower back.*

KID-16 Vital Centre

Virtues: This Energy Release Point allows one to get to the Heart of the Matter - to explore deeply within one's depths the imbalances of the physical, emotional, mental and spiritual bodies. Often these imbalances present themselves in the form of stomach ailments. Further examination holds that these stomach issues stem back to one's relationship with the feminine. Whether it is a personal relationship with our human mother, or whether it is the acceptance of one's own feminine nature (present in both males and females) or also one's perception of women in society and the value thereof. Simply put, there is a disconnection between our Selves and the Archetypal Divine Mother of the Birthing Feminine Matrix. Unblocking and activating this Energy Release Point allows us to explore these relationships and how we function with them, with this awareness, the flood gates open and a resurgence of new ideas and creativity flow and find their way into our consciousness. This flowing serves to heal our creative centre and through harmonization with the centre of the Divine Feminine Birthing Matrix one gains access to unlimited potential and possibilities of creation.

Disharmonies: *Blocked creativity; lack of vitality; exhaustion in the full body system; digestive disorders leading to depletion; dysfunctional relationship with mother and/or mothering roles; obsessive thinking; anxiety; emotional neediness; insecurity.*

KID-17 Accommodate, Deliberate and Trade / Accommodating Merchant

Virtues: This Energy Release Point metaphorically connects to where we are on our life journey and speaks to the point in the journey where fatigue and weariness can discourage the continuation on the path. It is here where we sit and re-structure, re-align and re-evaluate. This Energy Release Point is the point where we assess our inner qualities and our gifts, as well as the place where we evaluate the ability to assess the quality of our expression. It penetrates inwards to bring forth our unique Essence. Unblocking and activating this Energy Release Point allows us to find the value within, to bend and to be flexible. To be able to make changes within the journey and flow with Spirit. It allows us then to deliberate and trade, to evaluate our resources and know the quality of our worth. Much like the accommodating merchant who replenishes our supplies to continue the journey.

Disharmonies: *Inability to express feelings, especially deep sadness; weariness of life; internalized grief and melancholy. Physical manifestations of intestinal pain and abdominal fullness; no pleasure in eating.*

KID-18 Stone Border / Stone Gate

Virtues: This Energy Release Point speaks to the strength and permanency of the stones, rocks, and minerals. The mineral kingdom. The mineral kingdom is diverse. There is magnificence in the majestic peaks of the mountains and yet there is simplicity in the silhouettes of these same mountains and boulders. There is mysteriousness in the stones found in the watery depths of streams, rivers and brooks. The mineral kingdom continues to stir our creative senses when we observe the glittering sparkle when they are faceted into gems. Minerals are strength. They are foundational, solid and enduring. Minerals and rocks may be broken however they cannot be forced into being something that they are not. Minerals are an integral part of the earth, therefore unblocking and activating this Energy Release Point also opens us up to the Earth Mother. The source of nourishment, health, and the building blocks of the physicality. Minerals are therefore an integral part of us. This Energy Release Point resonates deeply to the sound vibration of the Earth helping us to receive and process nourishment in order to digest food and life experiences. From this Point, movement is empowered from the strength and solidity of the stone, transcending fears that would otherwise leave us stone cold or hardened like stone.

Disharmonies: *Pattern of finding obstacles on the path in all of our actions; being hardened by life experiences. Physical manifestations present as coldness within; abdominal pain and hardness; stomach spasms; digestive issues and infertility.*

KID-19 Free Passage Within the Inner Capital

Virtues: This Energy Release Point is a point of entry into the palace of tranquility found within the busy metropolis. A city can be rich in many things of beauty and elegance such as art, education, architecture, food, music and theatre; all that which creates culture. A city can also hold distractions of busy-ness, noise, clandestine and questionable behaviours, social barriers, violence and fear. With all the stimulation that a city brings, it can be challenging to find peace and tranquility. Unblocking and activating this Energy Release Point reminds us that we have a choice. The passageway to tranquility within is free and we can find liberty and freedom when we choose to dissolve the illusion of the importance of the material world. This Energy Release Point provides a passageway leading deep inside to the inner chambers of the heart where balance and harmony reign and tranquility is a natural state. This passageway restores peace from the heart to the mind.

Disharmonies: *Hypersensitivity to the environment; sensory conges-tion; tension; stress; obsessive thinking; worry; fear; overwhelm due to excess stimulation.*

KID-20 Through the Valley

Virtues: This Energy Release Point lends strength and builds the support-ive energy of having a safe haven - the place of protection and comfort when dealing with darkness. It brings back to awareness the knowing of being connected to the Divine. Once this awareness takes root in con-sciousness, the feelings of love and support can be embraced while under-going the experience known as the "Dark night of the Soul". Embracing the love and support of the spiritual realm allows for the return to balance and calm so that one can once more see the Light. Unblocking and acti-vating this Energy Release Point is similar to shining luminosity into the darkness within, in order to clear the path to transcendence and higher consciousness. This is done through the cleansing of fear and other dark emotions by actively confronting and healing the pain. It strengthens faith and trust in a higher power to know that all will be well and empowers the ability to release the old and emerge into the light to be reborn and made new.

Disharmonies: *Fear; disconnection; loneliness; isolation; acute suffering; panic attacks.*

KID-21 The Dark Hidden Secret Gate

Virtues: This Energy Release Point is the entrance to a dark hidden secret gate. It brings one to an opening into the darkness. It is also to understand that there cannot be a full understanding of darkness without having the experience of seeing light. Also, it is to understand that within even the darkest places, such as the vastness of a night sky with a new moon there are still stars that shine. Within the darkness there is light, within light there is darkness. Walking through the dark gate into the place where emotions and experiences are hidden and forgotten in secrecy allows for the empowerment to transcend fear and to promote flow to joy and freedom. Dark Hidden Secret Gate symbolizes the entry to the burial ground of emperor- the mausoleums, a place of great reverence. Likewise going inwards to face one's darkness, pain and fear is a journey of healing with reverence. Unblocking and activating this Energy Release Point allows for going into the underworld, into the depths of the heart and to bring illumination. It is introspection, and faith in trusting one's inner knowing and wisdom.

Disharmonies: *Inability to face fears; escapism behaviour; searching for external sources for reassurance; over-dependent on others, emotional co-dependence. Physical manifestations of bloating; heaviness; digestive issues.*

KID-22 Walking on the Verandah

Virtues: This Energy Release Point promotes the sense of satisfaction found upon the completion of a stage of the journey. It is in this place that one can evaluate the progress of the journey. To contemplate, to relax and refuel one's energy before proceeding onwards. It is having arrived at the realization that true joy is the positive effect of having devotion to a pur-poseful life. Once the realization is made, it is then to discover and receive heavenly inspiration as to the next steps on the forward journey. Fears are transcended and replaced by joy and ebullience. Feelings of renewal and refreshment surge forward. Unblocking and activating this Energy Release Point replenishes vitality for living. It renews joy, optimism and enthusiasm in the heart. Heavenly inspiration communicates purpose to the Soul and the Heart forces spark passion and positive action.

Disharmonies: *Depletion due to the pursuit of happiness resulting in empty pleasures; lack of direction and purpose; being weighed down by mundanity; experiencing exhaustion after a long struggle; slow recovery from illness or injury.*

KID-23 Soul Seal of Spirit

Virtues: This Energy Release Point speaks to the identity of who we are. The opening of this seal unlocks the information of why we are here. It is much like receiving and opening an important document that has travelled through the passage of time and lifetimes of the Soul. A document that has been sealed with the print of the Creative Force and our individual I AM presence. It is an agreement which receives utmost reverence and honour. This is the Essence of one's identity. Upon this understanding of one's absolute sacredness of Being, it is absolutely appropriate to demand of oneself love, honour and respect and by so doing, receive the same from others. In Ancient times it was understood that Divine Energy grants us life. Therefore the ability to think, move and take action was gratefully received as a way to express the Divine in action through physicality. Humanity walked the earth, connecting with the physical elements for physical nurturance while remaining connected to the heavenly spirit. Through the passageway of the heart, one could live their life in a meaningful, purposeful way, manifesting and activating their unlimited potential. Unblocking and activating this Energy Release Point connects to and opens the seal to one's divinity where inner wisdom of the heart knows the who and the why of the individual's existence.

Disharmonies: *Feeling lost in life direction; isolation; lack of authority; doormat syndrome; not feeling like oneself; fear or disconnected as a result of entity invasion or possession.**

*Should this be the disharmony it is important to release and clear the lower aspect, dark aspect, entity or possessive force from the field and whole body systems, as well as any residual energy of the preceding before activating and unblocking this Energy Release Point.

KID-24 Spirit Wasteland / Spirit Burial Ground / Spirit Wall

Virtues: This Energy Release Point enhances the ability of making change in the world. It activates one's power and helps to manifest potential. It is to harness all potential with the realization that one has the ability to create and manifest using the Universal Laws. What is more is that the creation and manifestation unfolds with seemingly little effort. Unblocking and activating this Energy Release Point helps to unearth the Spirit within so that the Soul can express through the physical vehicle in a more passionate way. Metaphorically speaking, activating this Energy Release Point is similar to bringing water to a parched, barren land, so that life may spring up through the cracks and flourish, renewed by the resilience of Spirit.

Disharmonies: *Disconnection from Source and Spirit; feeling as though life has been wasted or that life is in ruins; building walls of protection around the heart which in turn leads to isolation and retreat from society; physical exhaustion and depletion.*

KID- 25 Spirit Storehouse

Virtues: This Energy Release Point provides access to the spirit of the Heart. The spirit of the Heart is that of wisdom, inner knowing, inner authority, self respect and trust. It is an infinite resource that is always available. It is the spirit of the Heart in the shelter of the inner heart chamber, the resonance to the I AM Presence. The I AM Presence has absolute knowing and trust in the Divine, and from this comes the strength to conquer anything. To move through obstacles with the will, empowered by Divine Will, to carry on. Unblocking and activating this Energy Release Point helps to remove any shelter or walls that have been erected to protect the Heart from disrespect all while strengthening the love of Self so that the conditions for the reception of anything less than love cannot exist.

Disharmonies: *Doormat syndrome; disempowerment; fear of intimacy; caught in a cycle of abuse, disrespect and/or violence.*

KID-26 Within the Centre of Elegance

Virtues: This Energy Release Point assists in removing stains or tarnish from our original nature or Essence. It is much in the same way that a jeweller removes tarnish from a piece of precious metal and jewels. Our original nature, our Essence is a jewel buried within our depths. It is something precious - more precious than the purest diamond, for it is the concept of an entrusted sacredness. This is a priceless jewel has been invested within us by Heaven and our Divine Self at the moment of our conception. Recognizing ourselves as this priceless jewel we begin to recognize the jewel within others, and from this we begin to recognize the beauty within all. Furthermore, the recognition of beauty inspires the creation of beauty. The creation of beauty through art forms such as poetry, music and visual art become an experience of devotion. We are a point of light within the mind of the All and from the Divine Mind, comes Divine Will. When our little wills connect with Divine Will, purpose and light integrate. Purpose driven devotional expression manifests as a way of living and therefore, we can rule our lives with ease and grace through all experiences and times of great change and transition. Unblocking and activating this Energy Release Point ensures that the light that we embrace and live allows for our virtues to shine forth effortlessly. In this way, unconditional love can flow with ease to and from the Heart.

Disharmonies: *Negativity; negative perceptions of life brought on by shock and trauma; obscurity of both perception and manifestation of our innate* *beauty; inability to connect to our creative gifts; disconnection from the heart; living only in the mind.*

KID-27 Treasury of Source

Virtues: This Energy Release Point is an interface which conducts messages of wisdom, enthusiasm and creativity from the great treasury of Source. A resource of infinite vitality. Unblocking and activating this Energy Release Point activates a conduit of transportation. In the transportation process, this energy from Source is alchemically transformed into inspiration with a desire. It is the fuel of desire which then proceeds to create dynamic positive action. Furthermore, anxiety and fear are transformed into breath and inner tranquility, so that actions unfold from a strong centre of vital energy.

Disharmonies: *Anxiety; fear; fatigue and exhaustion from over striving.*

Portraits of the Energy Release
Points for the Energy Release
Channel of the Pericardium

P-1 Heavenly Pond

Virtues: This Energy Release Point evokes the image of a sacred and tranquil pond in which one can bathe in the purity of the Holy Spirit. A place where one comes in order to be cleansed and healed from the shadows and scars of life experiences. Bathing here serves to remind us that just as a pond is part of a larger living water - we too - our Essence is part of a larger bigger Essence - that of the I AM - God Presence. Unblocking and activating this Energy Release Point restores, calms and renews the qualities of purity and love. It has the ability to transport beyond the limitations of time and space to a boundless time and space of a larger, vast heavenly relationship. It is truly a renewal of the memory of safety that is untouched by life experiences. The memory of our heart as being a place of ultimate safety - free from the shadows of negativity that are imprinted upon us by the planetary consciousness of humanity's accumulated experiences.

Disharmonies: *Lack of compassion towards self and others; accumulated pain and betrayal which blocks intimacy; disempowerment; fear of embracing life.*

P-2 Heavenly Spring / Heavenly Warmth / Heaven's Revival

Virtues: This Energy Release Point empowers feelings of safety. The safety that is remembered from the time before life experience. It is this feeling of safety that allows for the heart to open and be receptive to intimacy. It is this same feeling of safety that breaks down the walls of self-protection and initiates the movement and action to a place of positive vulnerability. Unblocking and activating this Energy Release Point allows forward motion in the world, with the ability to apply the lessons learned from having had a painful experience. This assists one to initiate action in the world by being able to flow strength and compassion from the healed heart. It empowers the ability to move from pain to trust, from trust to embracing life and from embracing life to being filled with compassion and joy.

Disharmonies: *Cold-heartedness; bitterness; overly protective of space; barriers; fear of intimacy.*

P-3 Crooked Marsh

Virtues: This Energy Release Point facilitates open-hearted sharing, trust, fortitude and contemplation. It allows one to strengthen the ability to set healthy and appropriate boundaries especially in intimate relationships. Unblocking and activating this Energy Release Point amplifies the feeling of joy when experiencing intimate connection within a loving setting.

Disharmonies: *Inappropriate boundaries in regards to sexual relationships; feelings of betrayal; nervousness and anxiety; impulsiveness in regards to intimate relationships; lack of joy; projection of past pain in present relationships.*

P-4 Gate of Energy Reserves

Virtues: This Energy Release Point refers to a gate or a door which is not secure. It can also refer to a key to open the gate or a key to opening a portal. However daunting it is to open a gate or portal, for fear of what is on the other side, it is vitally important to do so. This particular opening is to plunge deeply into issues that are focused particularly around the family, a clan or a group with whom one strongly identifies. This plunging into the depths of pain allows for the breaking through of blockages caused from past heartbreaks and betrayals. Unblocking and activating this Energy Release Point transforms painful blocks for the creation of peace and serenity in the heart, mind and soul. It is this transformation that ultimately heals the mental/emotional and physical body. The gate then becomes free and can open and close with ease as deemed appropriate. Stability, security and harmony are restored to the body as more and more feelings of anger and sadness are consciously transformed into feelings of tenderness. Through Gate of Energy Reserves one realizes that it is safe to love ourselves and others.

Disharmonies: *Shutting oneself off from intimacy and warmth; dysfunctional family issues; feelings of anger; unresolved issues of painful separations; beliefs that intimacy or any heart relationship is not safe.*

P-5 The Intermediary / Ghost Road

Virtues: This Energy Release Point empowers the heart to receive and let go especially in regards to grief stemming from lost love and betrayal. It provides for an alchemical transformation of the mundane consciousness and over-personalization of one's pain and attachment. The alchemy is precisely a shift in consciousness as the world and life experience is transformed into gold. It is to open to non-attached awareness. From this shifted awareness we open ourselves to loving exchange by the virtue of gratitude. As Ghost Road implies, we release the shadow aspect of pain of lost loves, unrequited loves, possessive loves, in short, all the "ghosts" of past loves in order to move forward and bring in the higher love potential of a new sacred union.

Disharmonies: *Grief and longing for lost love, unattained love, unrequited love; inappropriate holding on to relationships which have ended; shutting of the heart from intimate connection; attracting dysfunctional relationships; repeating a pattern of unfulfilling relationships; sabotaging good relationships; inability to move on towards new relationships because of past pain; perfectionism and judgment resulting in separation in new relationships; having attachments and desires associated with past loves.*

P-6 Inner Frontier Gate / Inner Palace Gate

Virtues: This Energy Release Point embodies our journey into our hearts - the frontier and unexplored territory known as the borderlands. The journey into this transition zone cannot help but create transformation - for in the act of undertaking the journey itself one is transformed through the encounter of the unknown. As a gate point, one is empowered to come and go at will understanding the appropriate boundaries in relation to the sanctity of the Heart and sharing oneself with others. Qualities of compassion, connection, warmth and Light are accessed and bring the perseverance to proceed onward with the journey. Unlocking the gate to this inner heart space signifies a profound turning point for the one willing to pass through and transform pain and hurt into blessings of peace and calmness. Unblocking and activating this Energy Release Point can assist in calming the Self from the trauma of betrayal from intimacy, rape, incest or divorce.

Disharmonies: *Closing the heart in self protection from the pain of intimacy; projecting old pain onto the present; feelings of being stabbed or shot in the heart due to betrayal or painful separations.*

P-7 Great Tomb / Ghost Heart

Virtues: Many civilizations honour the deceased by burial in designated areas of a village. These places are set aside with reverence. They create a sacred space to honour those who have transitioned from the physical plane of existence. Often times, these places would also serve as sites for celebrations. In celebrating the life and the enrichments of those who have gone before, prosperity and gifts continue for the future generations. Each life is sacred. A life has jewels from experience, and from the jewel great treasure is revealed. From the heart of Great Tomb comes strength, stability and support to assist in the present life journey. Unblocking and activating this Energy Release Point helps one to connect consciously with the gifts of our ancestors. It assists in focusing the energies, the insights and the visions with calmness and wisdom, so that we can create and embrace a life of joy. It is to follow therefore, that when one is in this vibration of joy, strength and support, that hearts can open more easily to relationships of nurturance and intimacy. The alternate name of this Energy Release Point - Ghost Heart - speaks to the facility that one may become obsessed with the inglorious aspects of death, the dark, the macabre, the painful and suffering. By associating with these lower aspects, sympathetic merging with discarnate beings can result. Many of these discarnate beings are bound to the Earth plane by their own attachments to pain and suffering. Unblocking and activating this Energy Release Point in this context, is therefore very useful in the alchemical process of transmutation of suffering and thereby releases entity possession, obsessive thoughts and obsessive, compulsive behaviours.

Disharmonies: *Insecurity; anxiety; mental instabilities; overly porous aura.*

P-8 Palace of Weariness / Ghost Road

Virtues: This Energy Release Point connects to the inner chambers of the heart. These inner chambers contain a soft lamp and illuminating presence. This illumination exemplifies the quality of Soul essence as it is always present despite even the most trying times of darkness. The strength of this light has influence - it can vanquish darkness, psychic infiltration of entities, ghosts or possessions. It has the ability to illuminate all matters of shadow and then reconnect with the Ultimate Source of Light and Life for all. Nourishing this light empowers the virtues of openness, warmth and safety. Protection that comes from a base of love guards and enhances one's light. Protection that comes from a base of fear, does not protect. Fear can be fed by entities, ghosts and possessive spirits and can fill one with paranoia, amplifying fear. Unblocking and activating this Energy Release Point connects one to the sacred inner chamber. It allows one to open the heart, it empowers courage to love and to live within the context of fulfillment and joy. Through joy and love, we can more fully embrace ourselves and others by the action of releasing the demons of the past.

Disharmonies: *Addictions (in particular lust and bliss); paranoia; fear; mania; depression; lack of joy; lack of will to live; weariness from life; pain of heartbreaks; closing the heart to oneness and intimacy.*

P-9 Rushing Into the Middle

Virtues: This Energy Release Point brings a surge of strength to our central core, unleashing vitality to energize our full body systems. It brings forth spontaneity, flow, motivation and encouragement. It fuels desire, prompting us to seize the day and burst into action. These desires can include relationships, creative pursuits and life dreams. Unblocking and activating this Energy Release Point empowers vitality, energy, motivation and drive as well as trust, tenderness and intimacy. It inspires us to zone in and focus on our vision. It is to see the target, aim purposefully and attain the goal. This Energy Release Point harmonizes the surge of impetuous energy with discernment so that the goal in pursuit is one that is beneficial to our highest good. It balances the flow of energy for creative pursuits and life dreams so that they can be directed by heart-inspired logic. It creates a moderating energy so that intimacy can function in a healthy, balanced way.

Disharmonies: *Lack of perspective; dysfunctional relationships; distrust; burnout from overuse of creative forces; sexual addictions.*

Portraits of the Energy Release
Points for the Energy Release
Channel of the Three Elixir Fields

TH-1 Rushing the Frontier Gate

Virtues: This Energy Release Point assists in the ability to speak clearly and authentically. It facilitates the connection to the warm fires of the heart, in order to bring forward this warmth as a virtue of creating welcome within a social context. It further assists one to receive inspiration and joy during social exchanges. As a Frontier Gate, this Energy Release Point allows us to create healthy boundaries, so that social exchanges occur in a balanced way, with a defining perimeter. A perimeter that allows for healthy and positive interaction where everyone benefits from uplifting exchanges. This healthy boundary manifests on the physical plane as a healthy immune system - protecting us from viruses, bacteria and toxicity. Manifesting on the social level, the perimeter of our boundary is determined by what degree our vibrations of spirit and light can extend into the world while being able to hold its integrity. The outermost layer of ourselves, similar to the vastness of the unknown frontier, represents the outermost layer of our consciousness. We become more aware of where we and our consciousness end and where the unknown outer world begins. We become a grounded presence within ourselves and less affected by those whose Essence and core are incongruent to our own. We are able to seek and find those who inspire and kindle joyful resonance within our hearts. Activating this Energy Release Point empowers us to extend ourselves into an expansive world and universe in an inspired yet protected way.

Disharmonies: *Rigidity; coldness; numbness; emotional detachment; lack of sensitivity; inability to receive or appreciate the quality of incoming ideas; weakened immune system.*

TH-2 The Gateway of Outer Harmony

Virtues: This Energy Release Point is the gateway of harmonization between our inner world and our outer world. This gateway connects with the ninth part of both our vertical and horizontal, masculine and feminine energy fields. This ninth part of the field is called the Environmental Part and governs what the Ego (physical consciousness) needs to learn in order to feel its surroundings as well as the energies of the environment. From its perceptions it learns to discern what is beneficial or not beneficial for itself. It is this discernment that assists in the appropriate response. This principle also applies to the environment inside the physical body where imbalances can manifest. These manifestations can be attracted through thoughts, emotions and beliefs. This Energy Release Point is a transformational gateway allowing for the releasing, balancing and harmonizing of the environment. Unblocking and activating this Energy Release Point ensures that the gateway is moving easily so that joy, love, sharing and companionship flow both inwardly and outwardly. The world as well as life's experiences fill us with awe, the beauty fills us with wonderment and peace. It allows for discernment and clarity; therefore a support for the True Self. Once we allow this connection to our core, we can feel the depth of our Essence and trust that through healthy relationships (with self and with others) the beautiful Soul nature may be shared with the World.

Disharmonies: *Aloofness; withdrawal; isolation; over-sensitivity to the environment; compromised immunity; compromised integrity.*

TH-3 Middle Islet

Virtues: This Energy Release Point empowers vision as we turn toward the horizon. A horizon filled with expansiveness, freshness and beauty. It is to bring your Being into a state of centre and equilibrium on both the physical and mental/emotional planes. This allows for the ideal conditions in the receptivity of vision as transmitted from the higher spiritual planes. Energy centres of the senses such as in the eyes and nose become optimum as these are strengthened, stimulated and ameliorated. This fine tuning of the senses assists in empowering accurate perceptions of reality. From this centre, clarity of plans, decisions and goals can be made and brought more easily into fruition. Themes of birth, growth and hope begin to manifest with a renewal of optimism and vitality. On a physical level, activation of this Energy Release Point stimulates the elimination of toxins so that the body's self healing abilities are activated and connections to sources of vitality are strengthened.

Disharmonies: *Fatigue and exhaustion; overwhelm; indecision and lack of clarity.*

TH-4 Pond Source / Source of Communications / Communications Network

Virtues: This Energy Release Point has a strong connection with water - water being the streaming network or communicator of the body through the physical structure of the water cells aquaporins. Aquaporins are microscopic network communicators which serve to harmonize the internal God Source messages with those of the environment of the physical body, emotional body, mental body and spiritual body. The ultimate goal is to re-establish order and alignment between the internal primary Divine source with the Macrocosm of the Divine Cosmic Source; Solar Source. It physically balances hot and cold of the body and emotionally dissolves the illusion of separation with the higher sun source power. When harmony is restored, one can more easily extend one's actions to be of service and connect to the human family and earthly life in a more enriched and meaningful way.

Disharmonies: *Overly protective barriers; isolation; cold hands and feet; antisocial behaviour; feeling cut off from inspiration; living in "hell".*

TH-5 Outer Frontier Gate

Virtues: As this is a gate Energy Release Point, it speaks to the importance of harmony between the known inner realms and the unknown outer realms. In order for one to safely navigate the unknown, the feelings of security, safety and connection to inner truth needs to be firmly established within so that it may translate with confidence to the exterior. This gate function also translates to the ease and confidence one feels to embrace living life and participating in the social network. To feel joy in the companionship with others is energizing for the Soul. Unblocking and activating this Energy Release Point allows for discernment of who we extend ourselves to and with whom we do not in accordance with our highest good and wellbeing.

Disharmonies: *To erect barriers towards others; to have dysfunctional boundaries within relationships; social alienation; avoidance of intimacy; embarrassment; feelings of shame; low vitality; premature aging; compromised immunity; extreme fluctuations in temperatures within the body. (For example Reynaud's syndrome, hot flashes)*

TH-6 Flying Tiger / Branched Ditch

Virtues: This Energy Release Point has the ability to harmonize overactive abundant strength and energy with the deep strength found within the internal core of the body. By balancing these two seemingly opposite expressions of energy, vitality can more easily flow through the physical body in a regulated steady way, thus alluding to the secondary name Branched Ditch. This Energy Release Point acts as a modulator. If energy is low, the Flying Tiger/Branched Ditch brings a burst of exuberant vitality to entrain the lower fires of the vitality centre to ignite and fuel the body. If vitality is overcharged and in a hyper state which cannot be sustained, Flying Tiger/Branched Ditch assists in smoothing and steadying the flow so that vitality is evenly distributed. Unblocking and activating this Energy Release Point will help clear the whole body system, detoxify and clear sluggishness so that vitality is harmonized and flows in a sustainable steady way.

Disharmonies: *Bursts of energy followed by the lows of exhaustion and sluggishness; boundary issues caused by excessive hyper energy; promiscuity.*

TH-7 Assembly of Ancestors

Virtues: This Energy Release Point mediates the influence of ancestral wisdom as imprinted within our DNA; our source of Essence and it's ability to radiate this wisdom by heaven's spirit - The Creative Force. In Ancient China, the metaphor is one which shows the meeting of the feudal princes at the summer court. Here, the virtue is to unite and integrate the functions of all the officials in the kingdom, the same way that a well functioning thermostat maintains the environment of a house. The kingdom and the house within the kingdom is symbolic of the temple of the physical vehicle. With the harmonic unification of each aspect of the body as well the alignment of Soul purpose and destiny with the will forces, one experiences greater physical and etheric vitality. This alignment of thought, word and action also brings added clarity to intention and vision, which burns off the residual negativity lingering from attachment to the mundane and negative ego. Added inspiration stimulates the growth of awareness of one's genetic and karmic connection. This awareness helps to realign with the wisdom and virtues of our ancestors and therefore strengthens our foundation for realizing potential and fulfilling destiny. Our inner light is expanded by our strength of purpose, Soul passion ignites from the direction of the heart of the kingdom, and radiates healing warmth and compassion.

Disharmonies: *Blocked by issues regarding over-identification with negative attributes of genetic or ethnic lineage; limiting our possibilities in our present moment by over-identification with concepts of who we are based on the past.*

TH-8 Connecting Interval / Communication Pass / Communication Gate

Virtues: This Energy Release Point allows for clarity of mind in regards to life experiences and relationships so that one can communicate. Effective communication is an essential component for co-operative manifestation. This Energy Release Point helps to discern what is important and of value for furthering one's purpose, and what is unnecessary and inessential. The ability to release the inessential is enhanced. This is especially valuable in situations where one is called upon to mediate and harmonize group work - for one then is more equipped and able to extract what is essential through compassionate wisdom. Unblocking and activating this Energy Release Point helps bring the quality of flow in co-operative group work as well as equanimity among the participants. The virtues of integrity and alignment, as well as sincerity in communication, is enhanced. In the sense of a connecting interval, it is to create the space for movement. This is exemplified by the movement of musical intervals, creating harmonious melody, leading to the harmonization of three important masculine qualities: the ability to sort and separate the essential from the extraneous; to release the extraneous and retain the essence of the indispensable; and finally to harmonize the preceding two qualities into rhythmic communication to the greater whole and manifest brilliant potential.

Disharmonies: *Inflexibility; iron-willed; inability to harmonize strength and power with tenderness and gentleness; bitterness; disdain.*

TH-9 Four Rivers

Virtues: This Energy Release Point creates the expansion of space and allows one to flow in flexible direction in all aspects of being. It strengthens and increases the ability to listen. It flows the energy of balanced communication and thereby creates a harmonious community and group life. Unblocking and activating this Energy Release Point allows for a healthy boundary, harmonious group consciousness, flexibility and inclusiveness.

Disharmonies: *Imbalanced communication; stubbornness; unwillingness to hear the ideas and opinions of others; inflexibility; intolerance; self-imposed isolation.*

TH-10 Heavenly Well

Virtues: This Energy Release Point assures congruency between our wisdom of what we need, our knowledge and awareness of our physical limitations and stamina, as well as what we accept as sources of nourishment to balance our needs. The awareness of these three aspects are vital for a balanced life - and can be seen on a physical level as having the balance of food, rest and activity. This Energy Release Point also goes a step further and serves to ensure the even distribution of this balanced energy throughout our entire being. It promotes the awareness of positive action in regards to healthy lifestyle choices. Living a balanced life brings regeneration, rejuvenation and connection with universal love and support. The ability to embrace a lifestyle of moderation, healthy connections with others, and joy is facilitated with more ease. Feelings of gratitude and satisfaction in regards to daily tasks are enriched.

Disharmonies: *Lack of support and nurturing (physically, emotionally, mentally and spiritually) during childhood. Separation consciousness and feeling cut off from spiritual support and guidance. Dissatisfaction; longing; neediness; inability to digest life experiences; promiscuity; lust; emotional burnout; instability and lack of desire.*

TH-11 Pure Cold Abyss

Virtues: This Energy Release Point has the ability to channel warmth throughout the body. It is a warmth that thaws and transforms coldness into a vibrant physical presence. Pure Cold Abyss creates and strengthens the circulation and flow of light throughout the body. It further assists in warming the heart to compassion and love. Unblocking and activating this Energy Release Point allows for healthy embodiment and compassion towards self and others. It brings vibrancy to the physical body and helps integrate physical sexuality with love and spirituality to further empower living fully in the moment.

Disharmonies: *Withdrawal resulting from trauma in life; the pattern of "burning others" in a relationship from the overstepping of boundaries; excessive sexuality as protection from opening our hearts in relationships; excessive sexual desires; withdrawal and retreat from intimate contact resulting from being previously hurt in relationships; lack of emotional warmth. Physical challenges can present as gynaecological disorders and sexual dysfunction for men.*

TH-12 Melting Into Relaxation of Joyful Happiness

Virtues: This Energy Release Point is a pathway to joyful transformation through the virtues of beauty and relaxation. To see the beauty in all things and allow for the easing into relaxation that appreciation and gratitude bring. Warming our hearts, mind and body to the beauty that surrounds and bathes us in feelings of well-being and serenity. In this vibration we are filled with warmth, comfort and light. Unblocking and activating this Energy Release Point brings us meaningful connection to all that is beautiful; the art and music of nature, the ability to reproduce beauty through our own artistic and creative expression as well as appreciation of the creations of others. It is to find serenity, peace and mindfulness in meditative artistic pursuits. To embrace beauty in all aspects of life as a way of increasing light absorption in order to hold the frequencies of love, joy and compassion in our Being.

Disharmonies: *Stress from overwork; creative blocks; depression; feelings of betrayal; emotional coldness; overly identified with personal appearances; promiscuity; inability to achieve orgasm.*

TH-13 Shoulder / Upper Arm Convergence

Virtues: This Energy Release Point renews the abilities of flexibility and reciprocity. It is the ability to perceive and be aware of many points of view in order to assess the next active step. It also allows for harmonious group consciousness, for the ability to listen and take in differing opinions and evaluate options and possible choices. With a flexible mind, the ability to respond to life's demands becomes more balanced. From a balanced perspective, leadership qualities develop and appropriate delegation of tasks to others are facilitated by inspiration and example. Unblocking and activating this Energy Release Point enhances the ability to respond, balances receptivity and cooperation by empowering the ability to give and receive the necessary support in service to others.

Disharmonies: *Inability to ask for assistance; difficulty in sharing tasks leading to overwhelm and inaction; blocked leadership potential; overly intense in leadership. Physically this can manifest in shoulder pain.*

TH-14 Shoulder Bone

Virtues: This Energy Release Point helps to strengthen the shoulder so that it can continue to carry its load. It transforms the negative aspect of "load" into action of joyful service - a joyful service stemming from an inner source of strength in its alignment to purpose. Unblocking and activating this Energy Release Point brings joyful energy, enthusiasm and involvement in life's tasks. It renews strength and vitality in direct relation to our alignment with purpose.

Disharmonies: *Physical manifestation of weariness and fatigue; pain in the shoulders; over-extending one's boundaries; sacrificial service; withdrawal from service due to ingratitude, apathy and selfishness.*

TH-15 Heavenly Crevice / Heavenly Healing

Virtues: This Energy Release Point empowers warmth in the shoulder to assist in extending our heart into the world. When this point is unblocked and activated, it allows for the visualization of what we would see as heaven as well as support this vision and our abilities in bringing this vision into physical manifestation. It is however, more a state of vibrational frequency than a place. When this state is achieved, one can listen, perceive and understand the promptings of the Heart. These Heart promptings speak particularly to our relationship to the masculine energy within, as well as our fathers, brothers and/or intimate partners. Unblocking and Activating this Energy Release Point provides a space of harmony, allowing for a strong flow of Spirit and great transformation.

Disharmonies: *Fear of intimacy and friendships; withdrawal from social engagement; physical manifestations of frozen shoulder; arthritis; pain and stiffness in the neck and arm.*

TH-16 Heavenly Window

Virtues: This Energy Release Point allows for a glimpse of our spiritual connection to the Creative Force as it comes to us through love and light. It brings insight into communication and interconnections within ourselves and others. Unblocking and activating this Energy Release Point empowers us to know our authenticity and truth so that our actions are motivated by conscious intentions. It allows for a compassionate light to shine into our depths so that our shadow aspects can integrate and be transformed to courageous right action.

Disharmonies: *Blocking the flow of spiritual consciousness; disconnection between the mental and emotional bodies; escapism behaviour; emotions that run hot or cold; inability to face true motives for one's actions. Physical manifestation of body being too warm or too cold in different regions simultaneously.*

TH-17 Screen of Wind

Virtues: Wind is a natural function of the environment and has a cleansing effect. Its nature is dual; it can move things in order to expose something else or it can wipe things clean and erase all traces. This Energy Release Point addresses the dual aspect of wind, as well as the ability of wind to be flexible both in strength and its direction. Ultimately, Screen of Wind assists in our ability to work through change and transformation free from the fear of exposure. With flexible thought and action, one becomes empowered in such a way that the opinions and judgments of others have little influence as to how one moves through life. Unblocking and activating this Energy Release Point manifests the ability to create a screen from wind. A screen of wind which protects from external influences and clears the whole body systems of all that which would have a negative effect. It stimulates our immune system and maintains stability within, regardless of the external influences or chaotic environment.

Disharmonies: *Physical symptoms and signs which change rapidly in an unpredictable pattern; erratic emotional state; tendency to gossip; strongly opinionated; inability to form judgments and opinions; overly influenced by others; fear of public exposure; anxiety; fear of public speaking; fear of stage appearances; fear of crowds; schizophrenia; overly concerned with the upkeep of appearances.*

TH-18 Regulate and Support the Body

Virtues: This Energy Release Point has the ability to harmonize and support all the Energy Release Channels and by so doing, brings warmth, love, compassion, clarity and nurturance to all aspects of Being. Unblocking and activating this Energy Release Point allows one to create space in the environment to nurture a lifestyle that promotes harmony, balance and calm. It is through this clarity, self-love and self nurturance that all aspects of health can be addressed. The physical vitality is regenerated, renewed and restored; the emotional body feels enriched with healthy relationships with self and with others; the mental body becomes calm, stable and focused; the spiritual body connects with Source and expresses its abundance of joy, love and compassion - fully embracing life on all levels as an expression of a Divine embodiment. With this understanding of the importance of being responsible for the harmonizing and self care of the body system, the realization of healthy boundaries is also essential. The ability to care for one's self assures the ability to look after others.

Disharmonies: *Emotional and/or mental fracturing; body spasms; fear; anxiety; panic disorder; heart palpitations; chaos; insomnia; control issues; extreme negative emotions and violence; need to be in control; starved for love and attention; chronic illness.*

TH-19 Skull Breathing

Virtues: This Energy Release point allows the skull to breathe in order to gently ease any constraints of the mind and spirit. It allows for the harmony of intellect with emotion and compassion. Unblocking and activating this

Energy Release Point brings more focus, clarity and understanding of how to effectively apply what one has learned from going through an experience. It helps one to connect to a higher perspective and it is from this higher perspective that Spirit can more freely communicate with oneself and with others.

Disharmonies: *Overly dry intellectualism; to be stuck in the head; bottled up; overuse of the mental processes; overly strong intellect devoid of compassion for oneself or others; lack of focus; inability to implement the learnings of life experiences; lack of practicality.*

TH-20 Angle Grandchild

Virtues: This Energy Release Point acts as the connecting link in the line of generations past, present and future. It bridges future generations with the past and vice versa. A grandchild presents as an extension of a genetic lineage, like an ending, yet a beginning at the same time in the endless circle of family and life. This bridge embodies the wisdom of the elders and of traditions bringing discernment of the jewels into the future. Hence, empowering accurate perception of truth and reality of the present day, incubating and bringing forward these seeds of wisdom to flower in the generation of the future. Harmonizing the ability to grasp, see and listen. Empowering the virtues of clarity, sorting and intuition.

Disharmonies: *Dysfunctional relationship with parents and elders or traditions and family culture; inability to perceive and extract the wisdom from life experience gleaned from the observation and recognition of family dysfunction; issues of blame; living in the past; false and/or cynical projection of the future.*

TH-21 Gateway of Listening

Virtues: This Energy Release Point connects the pathway of the ear to that of the heart empowering the virtues of deep listening. It is the connection to wisdom. In order to truly hear, the words must enter the heart. Truly listening with the heart allows for all the words to integrate and transform. The virtue of strength allows for the hearing of words of strength and encouragement. The virtue of wisdom hears the words of wisdom. Unblocking and activating this Energy Release Point allows for the penetration of Sacred words so that respect for truth develops.

Disharmonies: *Stubbornness; rigidity of mind; speaking more than listening; inability to find inner stillness; mind chatter.*

TH-22 Harmony Hollow

Virtues: This Energy Release Point stabilizes and quiets the mind, stopping it from further agitation and disturbing the Spirit. As the name suggests, it creates harmony and therefore releases energy that causes misperceptions in hearing and listening. Unblocking and activating this Energy Release Point clarifies what we observe and how we perceive truths and reality. It allows us to flow harmoniously "in tune" with life around us. Harmony Hollow creates peace and allows our inner environment to interface in alignment with the outer environment.

Disharmonies: *Miscommunication; distortions in perception and interpretation; mental confusion.*

TH-23 Silk Bamboo Hollow

Virtues: This beautiful Energy Release Point invokes the image of the bamboo plant. The bamboo plant is a marvel of nature. It is strong yet hollow and can bend in the wind without breaking. In a Taoist text of the 13th century - The Book of Balance and Harmony - a beautiful verse is written in homage to the quality of bamboo. It is through this text that one learns about resilience, strength and integrity. Resilient Strength means to interact with events directly, managing the world with adaptability. It means to manage the mind with flexibility and manage the body with calmness. One also learns about Inner Emptiness, which means to forget emotions in action, to forget thoughts in stillness, to forget the self when dealing with events and above all to forget things when adopting to change. All of the above brings empowering connection to our own core. Unblocking and activating this Energy Release Point connects us to our core, strengthens our integrity and empowers resilience, strength, flexibility, balance and harmony.

Disharmonies: *Failure to nourish ourselves; over-extension of ourselves; disconnection from our true Essence.*

Portraits of the Energy Release
Points for the Energy Release
Channel of the Gallbladder

GB-1 The Sun, Before the Pass

Virtues: This Energy Release Point empowers the ability to receive light that serves to bring clarity in our perception of vision. This particular light is a light of innocence, bringing the energy of childlike trust, where one feels supported and loved by spiritual beings as we begin the journey of life. It empowers decision making and strategic planning. It is the first point of the Gallbladder Energy Release Channel and therefore is symbolic of the first light of the first day of life. Light becomes a source of spiritual nourishment, and is available to us from our first breath onwards. This continual reception of light empowers the ability to move through passages of shadow and darkness, firm in the knowledge that light guides the way to goodness and benevolence. Unblocking and activating this Energy Release Point empowers discernment regarding the goodness of the inner nature of self, as well as bringing into clarity the vision of the Soul for the life journey. It serves to empower beneficial relationships with others. It is confidence, security and trust. It ensures the stability of alignment between our inner plan and our life events through accurate perception of our Soul's vision. As one trusts their inner knowledge and place within community, living in harmony becomes the natural state of being.

Disharmonies: *Instability due to the chaos of life events; frustration; being overcome by obstacles; irreconcilable differences between inner vision and what we see in the world; discouragement and discontent; relying too heavily on the advice of others; having an overly rigid, inflexible judgment on what is right or wrong; to see only one side of any given issue; intolerance; belligerence; inability to consider anyone else's point of view. Physically these imbalances can manifest as heart conditions such as a heart attack or stroke, dizziness, cataracts and glaucoma.*

GB-2 Hearing Laughter, After the Pass

Virtues: This Energy Release Point has the ability to dissipate anger and fear so that one can hear and understand the messages of the heart. It empowers listening to life so that one can honour the intuition as well as act in a benevolent manner. Laughter is the language of joy. Living in joy requires trusting in the process of life experiences. It is to listen to life in a way that attunes and restores original intentions as set out by the vision of the Soul. It is the ability to see ahead to potential obstacles and find creative resolution before the obstacle has the opportunity to manifest. It is to live with intention so that the Soul can realize it's purpose. Unblocking and activating this Energy Release Point re-aligns Soul vision through the heart. Joy is experienced and maintained so that one can flow smoothly through life's obstacles.

Disharmonies: *Clenching the jaw in order to block hearing; anger; frustration; workaholic tendencies; inability to relax; headaches; resentment; habitual need to be right.*

GB-3 Above the Pass / Guest Host Man / Easy Host / The Great Sun

Virtues: This Energy Release Point harmonizes and balances feminine and masculine energy so that the ability to receive and to discern what can be released is enhanced. It promotes the flow of the Law of Reciprocity. Symbolically, this Energy Release Point also speaks to the sacredness of the trilogy - the union and balancing of Heaven coming into our physical body through inspiration drawn from Heaven, Earth as the solid support and foundation, and Humanity, the physical body that hosts the interaction of Spirit (Heaven) and Earth (Matter). Unblocking and activating this Energy Release Point helps to realize one's sacredness. It brings to awareness that one is a facet of the Creative Force and as such, a living embodiment of Love. With this awareness, the ability to live and embrace life with joy is enhanced. The heart and hands of service flow in loving exchange as one opens to share and receive the gifts of self and of others.

Disharmonies: *Withholding and withdrawal from society; depression.*

GB-4 Loathsome Jaws / Fullness of Head

Virtues: This Energy Release Point provides perspective on life, especially in regards to one's relationship to anger and perceived conflicts. The unblocking and activation of this Energy Release Point assists in finding inner tranquility so that one may openly acknowledge and transform anger and conflict through clear verbal expression. Physically this Energy Release Point helps to unlock the jaw, so to speak, in order to reduce harshness in words and tension in the neck.

Disharmonies: *Repressed anger; self loathing; to detest or reject situations or people. Physical manifestations include TMJ, jaw tension and jaw pain.*

GB-5 Suspended Skull

Virtues: This Energy Release Point assists one in connecting to inner wisdom and clarity in decision making. This is especially helpful when one encounters opportunities in the present moment and choices are to be made. Opportunities are viewed as potential for growth and expansion. Unblocking and activating this Energy Release Point allows for the tapping into stored potential energy, which is then used to put actions in place. The clarity of structured goals come from the revelation of how the completed manifestation should look. Seeing it from the end result of accomplishment. Our physicality is the means by which the Creative Force can take action. We are connected to the Creative Force through our upper energy centres located at the top of our head. This stream of wisdom is then brought into our body, and through our body, we integrate wisdom with the heart. Our minds and heart work in congruence and our actions follow through in surety and clarity. The ability to step into this action is related in degree to our rootedness and grounding of Spirit in our body and, by extension, our Earth and physical world. It is of utmost importance, therefore, to be fully present in the body, for this allows for upright, straight forward, purposeful action. Ultimately we are harmonious with life and with vision borne of inspiration and wisdom.

Disharmonies: *Lack of clarity; indecision; deterioration of vision (physically and spiritually); impatience; anger.*

GB-6 Suspended Tuft / Suspended Hair

Virtues: The name of this Energy Release Point reflects the fact that where it is mapped on the physical body is revealed beneath a tuft of hair. This is a powerful Energy Release Point in that it intersects the Energy Release Channels of the Three Elixir Fields, the Stomach, and that of the Large Intestine. Therefore, by this very location it integrates the highest of qualities of the virtues of these channels. Unblocking and activating Suspended Tuft/Suspended Hair brings forth the release of blessings and fulfillment which have accumulated over time (the Law of Accumulated Good) and integrates these blessings of life experiences in all aspects of Being. With a renewed sense of fulfillment and completeness, combined with the virtue of grounding through harmonizing with nature, there comes an awareness of contentment. Further realization is that this state is found through the grace of simplicity.

Disharmonies: *Endless pursuit of happiness and contentment; over reliance on the exterior props of material or social status with the illusion of happiness; constant seeking.*

GB-7 The Maze of the Temples

Virtues: This Energy Release Point has a historical significance. A maze is a network of paths and hedges designed as a puzzle. It is meant to bewilder and confuse. A maze has been used to camouflage a secret hiding place with intricate shrubbery that twists and turns. The surprising nature of these paths requires flexibility to respond as the need presents. This Energy Release Point enables this flexibility. It brings forward the ability to be an agile quick thinker to solve the puzzle and to move in a new direction. In life's circumstances, it is often required that one be able to change plans mid way. The maze is also a metaphor for initiation, a symbolic return to the womb, a "death" leading to rebirth, the discovery of a spiritual centre. It is the process of self-discovery, movement through life which, at times, presents difficult choices. Anatomically, this Energy Release Point is located at the temples - a sensitive spot - close to our brain and mind. It connects one to a place filled with wisdom and intuition. Unblocking this Energy Release Point assists us to connect with our knowing. The knowing that can sense our way within the pathways and turns that the journey of life is taking us. No matter what situation we may find ourselves in, by connecting to our inner centre - our I AM Presence - we can always find our way.

Disharmonies: *Feeling lost; disoriented; disconnected from purpose, passion and our path; embroiled in darkness and not being able to see our way out; depression; stagnation; apathy; indecision; inflexible and head-strong; oppressed.*

GB-8 Flowing Valley

Virtues: This Energy Release Point is about following direction. To be straight forward and to the point in a way which is of benefit for all. It empowers perspective which brings clarity in the continuation of life's journey. Part of life's journey is to flow through the valleys. The valley opens to be filled with the warmth of the sun and nourished by the rains. Through the richness of the valley, one encounters depth and darkness as well as growth and vitality. By unblocking and activating this Energy Release Point one opens to receive the riches around us. This activation addresses our ability to follow the directives of our vision and purpose, despite the fears of the unknown aspect of where the journey leads.

Disharmonies: *Stubbornness; inability to recognize and receive the abundance around us; fear; aloofness; superiority; arrogance.*

GB-9 Celestial Hub / Celestial Crossroads

Virtues: The name of this Energy Release Point is in reference to a star. This star however, is in a very active place, a place of full cosmic force. This place has active, dynamic, immense energy that serves to fuel and direct the lifestream of the Being connected to it. Each lifestream in physicality has a direct connection to their star. This Celestial Hub is also called Celestial Crossroads in reference to the many directional energies which converge at this point. These many directions represent the many opportunities which present in life's journey. These are opportunities which are interconnected, beneficial and serve to support vision and destiny. Unblocking and activating this Energy Release Point helps to diffuse congestion from an over busy mind by infusing the state of calmness within the mind. This calmness relieves overwhelm brought on by excessive planning or decision making. It is then, through the state of calmness, that one can align with Cosmic vision and have clarity in decision making that is congruent with purpose. It allows one to sit at the crossroads of powerful momentum and choose direction. This alignment with purpose creates a conduit for a great pouring of energy that revitalizes the body and supports forthright action.

Disharmonies: *Overwhelm; migraine headaches; hypertension; dizziness; vertigo; seizures; indecision; stagnation and frustration.*

GB-10 Floating Pure White Energy

Virtues: This Energy Release Point provides connection to one's true authentic Self. The True Self which comes from the purity of white light of Source. This connection reminds the ego personality that it is more than just an individual. That a person is a part of a sacred wholeness, and within that concept comes the realization that life, the body and the actions that one takes, have a greater purpose. In this way, energy is focused in a positive way to not only help keep one afloat, but to actually rise above the mundane density and dullness of routine, in order to be an active co-creator with the directives of the Higher Self. Unblocking and activating this Energy Release Point unblocks the flow of pure energy from the stream of consciousness that serves to direct decisions coming from Soul Source. Through this Energy Release Point, one connects with the ease of being one's True Self, a True Self that is empowered by the knowledge of the simplicity of just Being. This realization is the power behind the manifestation of dreams with ease and harmonious flow.

Disharmonies: *To over-strive; perfectionism; obsession with details; to float aimlessly without clear direction or vision.*

GB-11 Receptivity Within the Feminine Space of the Mind

Virtues: This Energy Release Point frees the ears so that one becomes receptive and better able to listen and receive higher guidance and wisdom. In specific, this Energy Release Point unblocks and opens the conduits from the physical ears, which communicate and link with the sensory energy centres of the ears. It is how these conduits penetrate that our mind acquires knowledge. It is the open and receptive state of the feminine energy to receive, through emission of it's inner light, that awareness moves towards wisdom and illumination. It is a necessary process of the inner nature to draw into the softness of meditation in order to bring light and clarity to the life process. With renewed clarity, the ability to perceive reality is empowered. The ability to articulate one's desires is also empowered. Unblocking and activating this Energy Release Point allows for speaking to become clearer, so that the language itself, expresses the steps necessary for the manifestation of goals towards the fulfillment of Soul Vision. As goals are completed, life feels purposeful and feelings of joy and contentment emerge.

Disharmonies: *Physical affliction of the ears such as tinnitus; living in the mind and not the heart; lack of perspective; disconnection with reality; inability to cultivate tranquility and connect with one's inner nature; lack of insight; miscommunication.*

GB-12 Final Bone / Completion

Virtues: This Energy Release Point brings completion. Whether it be the completion of a journey or a phase of growth and transition, it brings forward the energy of a well earned pause. A time to sit and reflect. The location of this Energy Release Point is on the mastoid process, that is, the base of the skull on both the left and right sides. The energy release channel begins at the eyes where one receives the vision or the directives of the Soul. As the release channel journeys towards Final Bone/Completion, it comes to a place where one can rest and reflect on the Soul directives. Unblocking and activating this Energy Release Point brings an energy conducive to meditation so that one can rest and contemplate the journey, strategize solutions for resolution of, and energy for, fulfilling the necessary action to arrive at a satisfactory conclusion.

Disharmonies: *Dissatisfaction in regards to incomplete business (with regards to personal work, projects, relationships); to feel devitalized; worn out; overly rigid and structured point of view.*

GB-13 Root Spirit

Virtues: This Energy Release Point anchors Soul vision into the physical body so that it can flower into manifestation. When one is living one's vision, the full body system (physical, emotional, mental and spiritual) functions as a harmonious whole. This Energy Release Point stresses the importance of the emotional and mental body in the process of integration between the spiritual and physical bodies. All four bodies work together. It empowers the ability to see and plan the necessary steps to fulfillment of vision, by defining and setting clear goals for achievement of purpose. It empowers a purposeful, joy filled tenacity to continue forward. It is a metaphor of the tree. The tree's roots tap into the water of the earth and through alchemy, integrates the water with the sunlight captured within it's branches. This process transforms the basic elements of water, light and wood into a living form called a tree. Similar to the tree, the energy field of the human draws in living light energy of the solar forces and cycles it through the body to anchor it into the physicality through the energy centres. It is the visual imagery of a being, standing firmly rooted in the earth, with the arms outstretched to the heavens, firmly integrating into physicality supportive energies which nourish the qualities necessary for the manifestation of purpose. Unblocking and activating this Energy

Release Point transforms Soul vision into physical manifestation by strengthening the ability to be fully present and grounded in the physical body. It helps in the planning of goals by supporting conscious intention and coherent thinking. It shines clarity in the understanding of the manifestation process by showing the steps necessary to create the strong foundation - the roots - upon which the entire creation is to be supported.

Disharmonies: *Unfocused; disorganized communication; overwhelmed and frustrated by too many ideas.*

GB-14 Pure and Clear Masculine Energy

Virtues: This Energy Release Point accesses the portal of pure masculine energy allowing for a great outflow of vitality. This vitality creates the momentum needed for manifestation of physical action. The strength and power of vitality can be likened to the energy of the sun: life giving, pure, clear and powerful. Unblocking and activating this Energy Release Point brings the energy of a new day, the sunrise, a day of endless possibilities, which flow effortlessly from one action to the next. Pure, clear masculine energy empowers clarity of vision and humility in the full body systems, releasing dysfunctional emotions that blind us from seeing our Essential Self and living our vision.

Disharmonies: *Inability to take straight forward positive action; indecision and lack of clarity; antagonistic projection; jealousy; envy; anger; judgment and arrogance.*

GB-15 Head Directed by the Kindness of Tears

Virtues: This Energy Release Point allows one to rise above self judgment, judgment and condemnation from others and empowers the release of tears which come from acknowledging the pain and frustration of the Soul's experience of being blocked from fulfilling its purpose of incarnation. Unblocking and activating this Energy Release Point allows for the positive action towards goals and desires. It empowers kindness and compassion towards self which extends to benevolence towards others. It allows for the flow of compassionate healing tears which serve to soften the heart, allowing for the healing energy of the heart to release and transform pain. This is similar to spring snows and rains that bring the vibrance of growth and greening. Through the release of tears, one can more easily release the old thoughts and fears, the toxic memories and emotions blocked and fuelled by frustration, in order to move forward in clarity of perception as well as in joy. To take action that is in alignment with our True Self, free from judgment.

Disharmonies: *Frustration; self judgment; overly critical with oneself; misperception of reality; victim consciousness; to be on the point of crying however not able to flow the tears.*

GB-16 Windows of the Eyes / Arriving to Greatest Glory

Virtues: This Energy Release Point empowers one to aspire to the highest manifestation of potential as directed by the vision of one's Soul Blueprint. It is about moving forward on our journey through life's experiences, learning lessons along the way in continual forward motion. It is to see the path directly in front in a clear, unobstructed view, free from distractions seeking to divert from fulfillment of purpose. This clarity of vision is further empowered by developing compassion for oneself and others so that the virtue of compassion is amplified and exemplified by one's thoughts, speech and action. Unblocking and activating this Energy Release Point raises consciousness, sharpens discernment, empowers forgiveness of self and others so that wisdom from events and experiences, past and present, create a higher perspective and continually serve the growth and evolution of the Soul.

Disharmonies: *Victim consciousness; belief that life is hard, unfair or a struggle; needing to be right; attachments to future expectations; past regrets; inflexibility; self defined by who/what is our exterior: i.e: job, education, family and spouse; attachment to the old story; judgment of self; judgment of others; blame issues.*

GB-17 Upright Living

Virtues: This Energy Release Point lends its energy to support straight-forward action and an unbending attitude in alignment with truth and purpose. It empowers desire for illumination and self realization, and assists in structuring goals towards manifestation of living the Soul's vision. It promotes living in a way aligned with the true Essence of one's Divine Self. Unblocking and activating this Energy Release Point nourishes the vision of the True Self. It strengthens the ability to stay in truth, despite exterior influences, by increasing discernment. It develops the virtues of authenticity, integrity and benevolence, so that thought and intention are in alignment with exterior action.

Disharmonies: *Confusion and indecision about life direction; lack of commitment; inauthenticity; feelings of anger and frustration; easily persuaded.*

GB-18 Receiving Spirit

Virtues: This Energy Release Point amplifies the action of moving Spirit from the body, to the heart, and to the mind, in order to connect with Higher Mind and then flow back down into the body. This action, once established, serves to magnetize Spiritual energy and connection to Ascended Beings of Light. It is amplification of prayer, ceremony, reverence and devotion. Unblocking and activating this Energy Release Point allows for the activation of the Spiritual interface, an interface which energizes our full body system to conscious awareness of our nature, our Essence and our purpose. It firmly supports the growth of our potential in co-creation with universal energy and cosmic forces. It strengthens sensitivity, empathetic receptivity and compassion, flowing these qualities to the external and blessing all those who are touched by its healing energy.

Disharmonies: *Spiritual pride; aloofness; insensitivity; lack of perception for consequences of actions; disconnect; illusion of spiritual superiority fed by false light; the perpetual seeker/spiritual junkie.*

GB-19 Vastness of the Brain

Virtues: This Energy Release Point allows for the thinking mind to open and expand so that it may move into emptiness. In the state of emptiness, the ability of the thinking function to receive inspiration from the Infinite Mind is enhanced. In this way, thoughts flow from the Infinite Mind to the mind, and manifestation of these thoughts can be guided from the Heart centre. Allowing the thinking mind this vast freedom of thought allows the pathway of Illumination to open, bringing vastness and expansion to the thought process. This empowers clarity of ideas, actions and emotions. Unblocking and activating this Energy Release Point has a direct result on the neurological physical functioning of the brain. It calms the nervous system so that higher thought and illumination is supported at the highest level, empowering an accurate perception of reality.

Disharmonies: *Mental disturbances; delusion; misperception of reality; impracticality; emotional constraint; anger; belligerence; inability to hear or understand messages from higher dimensional beings; headaches; tremors; tinnitus; inability to meditate.*

GB-20 Wind Pond

Virtues: This Energy Release Point helps in the navigation of life during times of chaos and upheaval. Wind brings change and during the process of change there is at times destruction and breakdown. Wind Pond has the ability to connect to the vibrant energy of wind and use that energy for the positive implementation of necessary action within the process of transformation and rebirth. It restores orientation, perspective and vibrant mental clarity. It helps one to make decisions and implement plans when faced with unpredictable life circumstances. This Energy Release Point unblocks the thinking life so that consciousness can be activated for higher activity. Higher thinking has the ability to penetrate deep into consciousness in order to reconnect to the essence of dreams and vision of the Soul. In this place of clarity, goals for the fulfillment of life purpose can be strategized and implemented into action. Unblocking and activating this Energy Release Point brings wakeful clarity. Clarity in the way of being keen and alert as though there are eyes on the back of the head. It is mindful and awake consciousness that can draw on the reservoir of wind energy to put life into action.

Disharmonies: *Inability to reconcile what we see in the world with our sense of self; remorse and regrets from the past; constantly changing plans and decisions; inability to deal with life's changing circumstances; sudden anger when needing to alter plans; inability to adapt to present circumstances due to inflexibility; indecisiveness and poor planning. Physically this can manifest as headaches; dizziness; sinus congestion; plugged ears and runny eyes.*

GB-21 Shoulder Well

Virtues: This Energy Release Point allows for the flow of communication from the Creative Force into our energy field and energy body in order to reach into our physical consciousness. It is through this communication that one can transform the pain of servitude and burden into joyous service. To be able to shoulder responsibilities in a successful and satisfactory way. A way which inspires benevolence, non-judgment and emotional flexibility. It is freedom from servitude. It teaches through example, the necessity of appropriate responses by honouring and respecting the needs of the self. Unblocking and activating this Energy Release Point provides insight into one's assessment of one's ability to respond. It allows for a higher perspective of joy to permeate the tasks that one needs to accomplish. Service to self and others become the expression of vibrant energy flowing from the regenerative properties of the Creative Force.

Disharmonies: *Judgmental attitudes; belligerence; inappropriate anger; constraint. Physically this can manifest as symptoms of tight shoulders and the inability to turn the head - leading to a limited perspective of life.*

GB-22 Humour Gate

Virtues: This Energy Release Point connects and activates the humours. The humours have been well known in the field of health, healing and sciences since the time of antiquity. The quality of the humours determines the quality of health and wellbeing. The common usage of the word "humour" is to mean the general disposition, the mood or feeling of absence or abundance of joy. This usage is derived from the ancient times when people believed that health and vitality went hand in hand with enjoyment, laughter and balanced living. Through the gift of mystics such as Hildegard von Bingen, the humours have been described as body fluids; the blood, hormones, lymph and metabolism that circulates throughout the body. When well balanced, the qualities of peace, discernment, perception, awareness and excellent health are amplified. The flow of the humours provide nourishment for regenerative cells, a strong autonomic nervous system, as well as empowering and regulation of the flow of the energy centres. This Energy Release Point opens the gate to the ever renewing wellspring of nourishment. It is a fountain that bubbles up to replenish and nourish the whole body system.

Disharmonies: *Withering of the body; aging; anger; judgment; devitalization.*

GB-23 Attached Tendon / Spirit Light

Virtues: This Energy Release Point assists the body, especially the limbs to flow smoothly and flexibly by strengthening the muscles and the tendons. These are essential qualities of strength that allow one to be able to move in all directions, free from encumbrances. It is a functional Energy Release Point in that one can compare its function to that of a well lubricated machine. A machine which runs smoothly, efficiently and easily in order to complete the task on hand. Healthy muscles and tendons empower growth and motivation by helping one to stand upright and connected to their path. As the alternate name Spirit Light suggests, it helps maintain communication with spiritual promptings and intuition of the heart along the driving forces of reason found in the gallbladder. In this way, it ensures that decisive action is based on forces that are aligned with wisdom and inner truth. Unblocking and activating this Energy Release Point strengthens the ability to bend and be flexible so that one navigates through life with ease, smoothness and freedom. It balances intuition and reason so that one respects the needs of the full body system. It eliminates the phenomena of mind over matter so that one knows when to take positive action and when to pause and listen for the next appropriate step.

Disharmonies: *Inflexibility in mind and/or body; frustration; resentment; paralysis; exhaustion; generalized weakness due to overextension of the will; symptoms of atrophy as the body breaks down.*

GB-24 Sun and Moon the Great Illuminators

Virtues: This Energy Release Point brings together two seemingly opposites: the Sun and the Moon. The Sun in it's brightness which represents outer illumination, that which brings light into the world and opens our sensory orifices to the outside, thus allowing us to perceive the world. The Moon represents the quality of light of the interior, inner illumination which closes the outer sensory orifices allowing one to look inside, into the depths of things and our Being. Unblocking and activating this Energy Release Point allows for the blending of these opposites into the unity of ALL - to the space of the One where all things are implicit within each other. This blending allows for higher perspective and discernment, the ability to see reality because of awareness of the balance between seemingly opposites. This Energy Release Point empowers perception of fundamental unity, releases judgments, strengthening harmony.

Disharmonies: *Extreme polarities such as optimism versus pessimism; seeing life only as good or as bad; lack of clarity; seeing only problems or finding only solutions for everyone else; inability to discern.*

GB-25 Capital Gate

Virtues: This Energy Release Point opens the gate to the wealth of the kingdom that is found within our Being. It is to access the wealth of our resources in order to create work that is fuelled by the growth and potential of the Soul Essence and brings ultimate fulfillment to life. It brings the energy of blossoming to the inner core and one feels the contentment of harmony and joy. The relationship between work and Soul purpose is a vital one. This Energy Release Point allows us to see within the depths and make connections between desire, talents and gifts so that our outer manifestation found in work can more fully express its alignment with Soul purpose. By so doing, it harmonizes the communications between the spiritual, mental, emotional and physical bodies so that work becomes an expression of inner calling. This communication is intricately supported within the integration of the full body system and nurtures the vital strength and well being of one's Being. When one connects to their purpose, one begins to desire, visualize and dream. This, in effect, grants permission for one to take the necessary action to live one's purpose. Dreams and desires are fulfilled. Abundance follows. The gate to wealth and resources opens and the perfect exchange of giving and receiving, as a natural outcome of conscious creation, is established. Unblocking and activating this Energy Release Point opens the gate to the motivating push to align with living purposefully. It allows us to draw on the wealth of our resources for vital energy. It brings the energy of freedom to pursue that which our Soul desires and strengthens the full body system.

Disharmonies: *Inability to feel satisfied; fatigue; weariness; confusion; indecision about life direction; lack of commitment or focus; fear; poverty consciousness; inability to recognize ones strengths, talents or gifts and how these same strengths, talents and gifts can be explored and developed to bring assistance to humanity.*

GB-26 Girdling Vessel of Vital Circulation

Virtues: This Energy Release Point activates forward motion which is steady and balanced, yet joyously enthusiastic. It embraces the sensory experiences of life to the fullest expression. Breathing in experiences, sights and sounds as well as tasting smelling and seeing the world in all it's gloriousness. It is through this Energy Release Point that one connects to the merging of the Soul with the physical vehicle. It creates expansion and regulates the flow of energy between the Cosmos and the Earth within the human body. Unblocking and activating this Energy Release Point is tantamount to lighting up an energy grid that powers up and creates a network of organization that puts life plans into action. Physically, this point is located on the waist, a place where traditionally money belts or coin purses as well as swords were carried. Symbolically, this refers to forward movement on the journey, free from fear, trusting that the necessary resources are in place and available for the adventure of life.

Disharmonies: *Stagnation caused by fear; immobility; paralysis; devitalization; physical manifestation of shingles.*

GB-27 Fifth Pivot

Virtues: This Energy Release Point has the meaning of being one of the five Energy Release Points that function as a pivot point. (ST- 25 Celestial Pivot, GB-28 Maintain the Way, DMD-5 Suspended Pivot, DMD-7 Balanced Central Pivot). Fifth Pivot anchors strength and balance within one's centre through periods of growth, great activity, transformation and change. It is a central pivot around which everything turns. A pivot is an immovable reference point of great calm and stability. It is to be in the centre of great action and activity, transformation and change. Unblocking and activating this Energy Release Point strengthens the ability to rotate flexibly around this central axis. It empowers a strong sense of self, which is balanced within group consciousness, so that one remains flexible and receptive in group work. It promotes decisiveness in thought, and flexibility in action, in order to bring into completion the manifestation of creative energy.

Disharmonies: *Inflexibility and rigidity of mind and body; low sense of self-worth; weak-willed; dysfunctional in group settings; over-attachment to personal will; easily overwhelmed by details; inability to formulate clear goals and plans.*

GB-28 Maintain the Way

Virtues: This Energy Release Point maintains the commitment to walk the path with clear intention and flowing flexibility. To walk the path is to trust in the fundamental unknowability of life and to have confidence to meet the unknown. To have clear commitment to walk the path, one needs clear connection to the will forces of the third energy centre. The third energy centre carries authentic power as derived from the alignment with Divine Will. It embodies the qualities of courage, faith, initiative, dependability, self-reliance and certainty. Walking the path magnetizes and radiates positive consciousness. This Energy Release Point is also a connecting point with the Horizontal Vessel of Guidance (The Belt Vessel). As such,it harmonizes and integrates all decisions and goals made to walk and live a balanced life. It serves to join together all disparate ideas and parts into a synthesized wholeness for purposeful action and mandalic consciousness. This living wholeness allows for the circulation of vital energy which fuels the generation of new ideas, further empowering flexibility within the birthing process to sift and sort through all the possibilities and move into appropriate directions for continual growth and manifestation. Unblocking and activating this Energy Release Point strengthens the commitment to walk the path. It sustains the energy of desire to become the feet, hands and heart of the Divine. Through being a living example of one who understands and lives "The Way", the ability for love and light to flow through the veil and touch the hearts and minds of humanity is magnified.

Disharmonies: *Feelings of constriction and restriction; inability to stay focused and on course; disempowerment; disconnected to purpose and* *vision; inability to follow through on intention. Physical manifestation of uterine problems; lower abdominal pain; lower back pain; unexplained water swellings; intestinal difficulties.*

GB-29 Dwelling in the Strength of the Bone

Virtues: This Energy Release Point empowers the feelings of protection by building the strength of the bones so that structure is maintained. It is here that strength gathers so that dynamic energy can be created. Wellsprings of energy are valuable resources for decision making, for once a decision is made, there must be energy in place for intentional action and concrete manifestation. Sometimes these actions are necessary break away actions. Break away action in that one needs to release themselves from self destructive patterns and lifestyles, or move away from limiting influences such as those found in family, friends or intimate relationships. This Energy Release Point not only finds the courage to follow one's own path and destiny, but assists in connecting to one's inner strength found within the bones. Unblocking and activating this Energy Release Point brings energy towards taking decisive action toward following the path of truth. It provides trust in knowing that the strength necessary to take the beginning steps is abundantly available. It brings centre and support to one's Being so that goals can be flexible within the virtue of positive structure. It further assists with the absolute knowing that one is loved, supported and protected by the spiritual world for the unfoldment of the Soul's journey.

Disharmonies: *Procrastination; inaction based on fear; doubt; confusion; inflexibility. Physical manifestation of disorders in the hip; lower back pain; atrophy in the legs.*

GB-30 Jumping Circle

Virtues: This Energy Release Point brings vibrant energy to spring into action with dynamism. To leap into life and put great plans into great action. It is the accumulated force of totality, perfection and completeness. The name Jumping Circle includes the ideas of permanence and dynamism for it is a continual flow of movement and cycle. The circle is the only geometric shape without division or point thereby representing the wholeness of the Cosmos. Interlocking circles are symbolic of unity. The circle is the most important and universal geometric symbol in mystical thought. Circles are also protective particularly in the world of fairies and folklore. Placing oneself within a circle assures protection from dark forces and negative influences. Unblocking and activating this Energy Release Point combines two principles: the ability to jump into action filled with dynamism and joy from the centre of a circle. A centre where one can be in union with the Cosmos and set clear focused goals that are aligned with Soul's intention. It is from this place of centre that one can formulate clear plans and take dynamic, proactive action with the assurance of Divine protection.

Disharmonies: *Stuck in the consciousness of "I should" or "I have to"; indecisiveness; fear of change; inflexibility. Physical manifestation of hip pain.*

GB-31 Market of the Winds

Virtues: This Energy Release Point brings together the qualities of the winds and it's observable effects. Winds are a way for planet Earth to sweep and purify the thought forms of fear which congest the atmosphere affecting humanity. This is seen as a cleansing process. The primary function of wind is to bring change and transformation; helping the natural world flow through seasonal change. The north wind blows cold and dry; the south wind brings warmth and moisture; the east wind brings snow and the west wind creates constant change. The Market of the Winds is a gathering place where all the qualities come together, empowering abundance and diversity of resources. These qualities are made accessible in order to help us through times of change, transition and growth. Unblocking and activating this Energy Release Point brings forward the energy of vitality and movement, assisting us to flow flexibly and gracefully. Empowering the ability to embrace change as a natural rhythm of life.

Disharmonies: *Numbness to life; numbness in the limbs; viewing life as pain; pain in the limbs; inflexibility; lack of movement; decreased range of motion in the lower back and legs; spasms; tremors; itching.*

GB-32 Middle of the Ditch

Virtues: This Energy Release Point evokes the image of the centre or middle of a waterway. A waterway contains elements of opposites. It can flow with rapidity or tranquility; it can reflect and sparkle in the light or absorb light into the darkness of its depths. Being in the centre of the waterway allows for the experience of observing opposites. Light and dark, warm and cold, movement and stagnation. In observation from the place of centre, one realizes the universal concept of unity and wholeness. For opposites are really one thing, on different points of a continuum. Moving along the continuum then becomes intentional and purposeful. Unblocking and activating this Energy Release Point strengthens the ability to sense direction upon the continuum of experiences. It allows for the observation of the spectrum of reality, reminding one that there is always choice and free will as to where one wishes to position themselves in the current of life.

Disharmonies: *Inability to stay in centre and make clear decisions; being embroiled in drama. Physical manifestations of pain, numbness and a decreased range of motion in the legs.*

GB-33 Passageway of Masculine Forces

Virtues: This Energy Release Point brings foundational masculine energy to forthright movement and action. Passageway of Masculine Forces creates the image of travelling through caverns of mountain passageways. There is form, strength and structure in the walls and the energy can move with swiftness and power. Should there be a fault in the structure of the walls, forward motion would be impeded. The walls would collapse much to the detriment of the traveller. It is in these instances that one stay flexible and seek a solution for either strengthening a structure, or for the removal of obstacles that interfere with attainment of one's goals. Unblocking and activating this Energy Release Point assures that the passageway for the flow of energy is unobstructed and clear. It empowers adaptability and flexibility within one's plans and goals. It balances the energy of giving and receiving by reducing rigidity.

Disharmonies: *Rigidity; inflexibility and the physical manifestation of knee pain.*

GB-34 Masculine Spring Mound

Virtues: This Energy Release Point empowers the ability to see things in a different perspective so that one may discover new ways in which to learn and grow. It helps to tap into the nourishing qualities of being firmly planted in the security of finding one's place on earth, and participating in life as an individual within a family or community. This Energy Release Point allows for the reception of energy from the fulfillment of positive actions done in service to others. It is precisely this interaction of open-hearted sharing between individuals that re-kindles the Soul's ability to energize and sustain the physical vitality of the body. Unblocking and activating this Energy Release Point allows for a branching out so that creative energy can flow towards healthy Soul growth. It facilitates the awareness of new points of view in the pursuit of goals and remove barriers for harmonious community consciousness.

Disharmonies: *Stuck in old patterns; resistance to change; fear; anger; anxiety; feelings of constraint; impulsiveness; being ungrounded; feelings of failure; frustration; impatience; inability to compromise in regards to cooperation within a group setting.*

GB-35 Masculine Intersection

Virtues: This Energy Release Point creates a network of harmony that unites the flow of masculine energy within the body. This fullness of flow can then direct power for the circulation of light force energy throughout the full body systems for well balanced growth. This Energy Release Point connects to the Masculine Vessel of Structure (Yang Wei Mai) whose function is to stabilize structure and to harmonize the body during times of change and periods of growth. In this way, it communicates the virtues of equilibrium and balance within the Universal Laws. Unblocking and activating this Energy Release Point promotes communication of energy with the masculine aspects of self. It balances distortions or vacillations of self within the context of the ability to harness and unify powerful masculine energy for action and completion of goals.

Disharmonies: *Distorted sense of self which erodes Soul expression; belief systems which undermine the ability to feel success or achievement; communication issues; strong ego with narcissism. Physical manifestation of knee inflammation; sciatic pain; pain and cold in the lower leg and foot; asthma and pain in the chest.*

GB-36 Outer Mound

Virtues: This Energy Release Point allows us to explore the unknown by enlarging the perspective of our reality. A mound or a hill is an elevated point upon which one can stand and observe the horizon in all directions. It is a place in which one receives the dream and vision and then sits in contemplation, filled with inspiration, as to the next decisive steps towards putting life in action. Unblocking and activating this Energy Release Point clears the panoramic scene before us. It illuminates potentials and possibilities, refreshing them from a higher perspective. It stimulates exciting changes, that are embraced with renewed vibrant vision, by simultaneously clearing out old patterns and toxic energies that drain us of our vitality and enthusiasm for living.

Disharmonies: *Dislike or fear of change; fear or aversion to wind; being entangled within energies of dark, brooding, congested and/or toxic emotions; bitterness; resentment physically manifesting as festering infections; excessive judgment of self and of others; excessive attachment to outcomes. First aid point for rabies.*

GB-37 Bright Clear Illumination

Virtues: This Energy Release Point brings together and harmonizes the relationship between the inner transcendental vision of the Soul and outer vision of what we see in physicality. When these two visions meet, clear communication between Soul Vision, strength of Will, and positive action towards manifestation of vision into physicality is enhanced. All vision is then viewed as a unified wholeness. The Light, emanating from the Divine Source can metaphorically be pictured as the Light of our Soul Essence. Our Soul is a piece of this light - the same radiance and energy but in a smaller way. This is similar to the way that the moon reflects the light of the sun. This Energy Release Point brings together these seemingly two opposites to a point of balance. Inner reflection shows that the Light is one and the same. Connecting in a conscious way to the Divine Light of Illumination and uniting it to Soul Vision serves to charge and strengthen Will forces of action. The Bright Clear Light of Illumination serves as a beacon to guide us through life. It brings clarity and facilitates discernment. Unblocking and activating this Energy Release Point allows for the integration and harmonizing outer and inner vision, all the while empowering the understanding that all things in manifested form and un-manifested form are one. As one, they are of our creation. Connecting with this energy allows one to see into Inner vision, have clear set goals and begin positive action towards positive manifestation.

Disharmonies: *Resentment; inaction; misperception of reality; rigidity with a tendency to only see one side of an issue; the inability to flow smoothly with life.*

GB-38 Supported by the Strength of Masculine Power

Virtues: This Energy Release Point serves as a pathway of light. It is similar to having a direct connection to the Sun. The Sun carries powerful energy at all times, however, the springtime Sun has a gentle warmth empowering a connection to the human heart. The human heart, when in harmony, has a fiery passion. When the human heart has experienced pain and discouragement, the fires of passion have withered to a spark - a mere shadow of its former brilliance. The connection to the Sun via this Energy Release Point awakens the sparks from their dormancy, and acts as a catalyst to encourage and activate the sparks in order to create growth and movement within the heart. Unblocking and activating this Energy Release Point creates a sustainable energy fuelled by the heat and the light of the Sun Source of Life. It supports and strengthens. It brings sun radiant forces of confidence and stability allowing us to open and flourish.

Disharmonies: *Inability to plan; lack of goals; lack of motivation to create a future; apathy; feeling of flatness; feeling stuck without desire to make a change.*

GB-39 Hanging Cup / Hanging Bell

Virtues: This Energy Release Point is a union point between the Energy Release Channels of the Gallbladder, the Stomach and the Urinary Bladder. As such, it will address underlying energetics which are foundational to the three and assist with their integration. As the name Hanging Cup suggests, one can visualize the symbolic representation of these three elements: a tree from which a bowl or goblet is suspended which is filled with water gathered from the rains. The tree represents the gallbladder (wood element) the bowl represents the stomach (earth element) and the rain water represents the urinary bladder (water element). The union and integration of these three elements assists in amplifying energy to fullness. Three in itself carries the dynamics of multiplication, development, growth and unfoldment. This Energy Release Point therefore conveys the energy of pure expression. Unblocking and activating this Energy Release Point fills the bowl with water from Source - the potential of all creation. The Earth element unites with water to bring forward nourishment to sustain the expression. The wood element is empowered with strength, stability and clarity to walk the path, fulfilling the steps required to manifest the Soul's vision and realize potential. As the alternate name Hanging Bell, we are also given the sound picture of a bell which tolls. The purpose of a bell is to call, to alert and to bring to attention, as well as to measure time.

Unblocking and activating this Energy Release Point in this sense, brings about an awakening, an inner realization, a call to connection with Spirit. To seek the pathway back to Source and to discover and walk a purpose filled life. Activating Hanging Bell with sound assists in drawing out any discordant energies that distract, seduce or divert from purpose. Removal of these distractions keep us safe, protected and on the path of destiny. This is similar to how ancient peoples tied bells upon the ankles of their children for their protection. (The physical location of this point is above the ankle.)

Disharmonies: *Lack of clarity; inability to manifest ideas into action; inflexibility leading to body stiffness and arthritic conditions; inability to stand on one's own two feet; anxiety; issues with the skeletal system; generalized weakness in the legs; inability to hear the call manifesting into tinnitus. Physical manifestation of multiple sclerosis.*

GB-40 Wilderness Mound of Ruins

Virtues: This Energy Release Point evokes the image of the wildness of unstructured growth that is observed with ruins and abandoned land. When one encounters a place of this nature, the imagination begins to stir visions of the land's future potential. Wilderness Mound of Ruins enhances the desire to make change in the world, through the realization of potential. It empowers perspective, to be able to see in all directions without obstruction. This Energy Release Point also serves in drawing our attention inwards to contemplate the effects of the destructive tendencies of humanity, and how as a humanity one can cooperatively work together to create a new form, a new structure where harmonious consciousness can thrive. Unblocking and activating this Energy Release Point strengthens benevolence. It brings wisdom gained from a higher perspective on where we have been, where we are and where we are going as a one humanity. It heightens appreciation and gratitude with the realization that personal opinions are never absolute, that there is room for creativity and value in the acceptance of the differences of others. Clarity of vision in regards to the external world becomes relative to our interpretations, judgments and belief systems, hence, harmonizing the relationship between the individual and humanity.

Disharmonies: *Being lost in the life journey; rigidity of thought; overly influenced by peers and/or family ties; for when a person cannot see the forest for the trees; feelings of malevolence towards others; prejudice; intolerance towards others; envy; feelings of discontent towards the accomplishments of others.*

GB-41 Near to Tears

Virtues: This Energy Release Point acknowledges the expressions of frustration and anger so that it can be released. The original pictogram of this Energy Release Point is that of a man on the edge of a cliff, signifying danger. This image, in itself, speaks to the importance of the healthy release of frustration and anger, so that a dangerous situation, either to oneself or to another, does not manifest. Near to Tears brings energy to the expression of healthy tears so that one can move forward, find courage, and make decisions that benefit the health of the Being and relationships with others. It assists in healing areas of darkness and shadows where repressed anger stews, waiting for the opportunity to burst forth. It brings healthy tears that function to relieve stress, especially when one is feeling frustrated and thwarted at every turn. This Energy Release Point is the master point in the Horizontal Vessel of Guidance (Girdle Vessel), which serves as an energetic belt to hold one together. Unblocking and activating this Energy Release Point assists in the release of stress so that one can feel reconnected to purposeful action towards Soul evolution and fulfillment of destiny.

Disharmonies: *Frustration; lack of fulfillment; stress; anger; hysterical behaviour.*

GB-42 Earth Five

Virtues: This Energy Release Point is a centre point, the expression of all potential. It is the convergence of four directions, and therefore, holds great power of the Creative Force. This power is the ability to realize freedom from a place of strength and centre. It is self empowerment. The number five is a perfect number, it is the expression of the Soul within the physical temple of the human body. It is the Human within the sacred trio of the Divine Masculine (Heaven), the Divine Feminine (Earth) as connected to heart's fire and passionate purpose. It is the middle between the number one, a beginning, and the number nine, a completion. It represents the life cycle - a beginning: movement from the spiritual world, into physical manifestation, where one walks the path of Self Realization to the completion. In music, the fifth represents openings, the freedom of expressed creativity, potential and endless possibilities. The number five is fearless adaptation, versatility and activity. Connecting with Soul vision, one strides confidently towards mastery of purpose, emotions and thought. This Energy Release Point is located where five toes meet the Earth. It is the ability to step into Mastery, to release frustration and to connect with the fifth dimension - a vibrational frequency where nothing less than the frequency of joy can exist. Realization of joy and freedom brings higher consciousness within one's physicality and reality. This higher, fifth dimensional consciousness embodies peace, harmony, joy and love on the Earth plane. Freedom is realized and Heaven on Earth becomes a reality. Unblocking and activating this Energy Release Point assists in connecting to the I AM Presence within the flames of the Heart. It assists in grounding in Spirit and walking a purpose filled life through positive connection with the Creative Force and Soul Vision.

Disharmonies: *Inability to connect with vision; inability to connect with inner hearing; lack of joy; lack of inspiration; physical foot pain; fatigue; over extending to others based on the inability to feel nourished from within; caught in a cycle of over giving without replenishment, depleting the ability* *to serve and nourish others. Physical manifestation in nursing mothers of insufficient breast milk.*

GB-43 Valiant Stream

Virtues: This Energy Release Point promotes the virtues of bravery and courage, and furthermore assists in directing this energy when one is called to be of service to others. It is to be able to respond to those in need, or to dedicate oneself to a cause or the rectifying of an injustice. It also provides the courage necessary to create a boundary between service and servitude. As the name Valiant Stream suggests, the energy of bravery and courage streams from an endless source of energy, empowering the qualities of perseverance, confidence and faith. This Energy Release Point therefore empowers the ability to flow with ease and grace around life's obstacles, with the knowledge that resources to fuel the reserves of energy required to complete one's task will be readily available. Unblocking and activating this Energy Release Point promotes flow in the process of Soul growth in relation to being of service, free from the sacrifice of the self. It provides vital energy needed to persevere in the fulfillment of goals regardless of the obstacles that are thrown in the path. Courage, bravery and chivalry serve for the benefit of the highest good for self and for others. Valiant Stream nourishes the energy needed to radiate tranquility and calming thoughts for healing distressful situations. It supports self-assertion and inspiration, and brings courage and bravery to stand up straight and tall as the situation demands.

Disharmonies: *Habitual rescuing behaviour; needing to be needed or wanted leading to devitalization; inflexibility; arrogance; lack of assertion; lack of inspiration; giving up in the face of challenges and obstacles; fear of success; over reliance on the intellect in the illusion of "trying to keep our head above water".*

GB-44 To Walk From a Place of Inner Light and Stillness

Virtues: This Energy Release Point gives quality to life and the quality of growth through life experience. The quality is defined as the ability to breath in inspiration and breath out that which doesn't serve growth and evolution. It is a quality unique to each, it is beauty and simplicity. Empowering simplicity, clarity, focus, inner dignity and value of Individual Essence. This empowerment allows for insight and deep understanding of the dual nature of One's Being. Unblocking and activating this Energy Release Point allows one to contemplate the inner self, where one's essential Light shines and where there is peace and tranquility. It allows us to be receptive to our true nature and move forward to realize our potential and manifest destiny.

Disharmonies: *Inflexibility; limited creativity; fear of letting go due to uncertainty as to what is essential and what is extraneous; indecisive; uncertain of life path; anger; self sabotage; resentment; blame of others in regards to not pursuing our path; despair; resignation; feelings of "what's the use?"; regrets; nightmares; sentences beginning with "I should have…."; insomnia.*

Portraits of the Energy Release
Points for the Energy Release
Channel of the Liver

LIV-1 Wellspring of Esteem and Sincerity

Virtues: This Energy Release Point connects to our Essence where one finds great esteem, sincerity, integrity, respect and honour. All qualities that are essential to deepen and strengthen the commitment to surrender. This Energy Release Point also helps one to be in alignment with inner vision, the inner vision that flows from the Creative Force. This alignment teaches the use of creative energy and empowers one to potentiate who one really is. From this state of being we honour ourselves and others. From wisdom one creates and shares that which benefits humanity, while remaining open to receive that which comes back in tenfold return. It is the realization that when one is in alignment with integrity, life in all aspects will have harmonious flow. Unblocking and activating this Energy Release Point gives strength, confidence and courage to reveal our true identity, set goals towards manifestation of vision with full trust that the path will be clearly marked and success ensured.

Disharmonies: *Problems related to flow and growth; feeling stuck; immobilized; stagnant and uncreative; lack of integrity; lack of commitment towards a spiritual path; laziness; attached to the material; lack of scruples; lack of moral compass; anger; low self esteem. Physical manifestation include gynaecological disorders; urinary problems; problems with the genitals.*

LIV-2 To Walk Between

Virtues: This Energy Release Point supports the alchemical process of growth. It transforms inspiration into positive action. It creates harmony within the Universal Law of Polarity, narrowing the pendulum swing between the poles of opposition, such as good versus bad, right versus wrong. This empowers the ability to flow in harmony and walk between the two extremes, carrying forth the energy of balance, peace and compassion for self and others. The energy of moderation in all things allows for flexibility in all areas of life. The 12th century mystic, St. Hildegard von Bingen embraced the idea of moderation as an essential component and guiding principle of behaviour for good health. In moderation, the imbalances of over-indulgence, addictions or severe aestheticism will not manifest. This Energy Release Point strengthens inner resolve, embraces hope as trust in the Divine outcome and empowers a bright vision for the future. Unblocking and activating this Energy Release Point brings peace and tranquility to the mind, joy to the heart and compassion to one's Being.

Disharmonies: *Inflexibility; belligerence; obsessive need to be right; the ends justify the means; tendency to give up in the face of challenge or adversity; polarization; burnout; despair; judgmental attitude; mindlessness; inability to think for oneself; overly influenced by others.*

LIV-3 Great Forging of Happy Calm

Virtues: This Energy Release Point connects to the energy of the Happy Wanderer - the Soul who experiences life, fully embracing all that comes with calmness and centred balance. This Soul walks firmly on the earth, planting one foot in front of the other in stability and security. It brings the knowledge that all life experiences accumulate into jewels of wisdom. This Soul energy realizes the importance of centre, and that balance comes from the ability to receive nourishment from within. Self care, self nurture, benevolence towards oneself serve to empower healthy boundaries through clear, loving communication. Unblocking and activating this Energy Release Point brings stability, vitality and balance. In this way, we are supported to carry out our plans and see them through to fruition, thus realizing our potential.

Disharmonies: *Anger; over striving; cynicism; belligerence; resentment; feeling stuck; projecting blame; inability to find creative solutions; inability to enjoy the fruits of labour; constant drive with the inability to relax and recuperate; conflict avoidance syndrome; digestive issues; throat issues; feeling burdened.*

LIV-4 Middle Seal

Virtues: This Energy Release Point is beneficial for strengthening identity and empowering the recognition of self confidence. It strengthens the ability to believe in one self and in one's ideas. It is the strength of this belief that assists in bringing the Life Plan into action. This Life Plan is embedded upon us at the time of our conception. It is the seal of the Divine Blueprint, the sacrament which makes our life precious, for the physical, emotional, mental and spiritual bodies. It constitutes the foundation of self-worth, self-esteem, and value of our Essence. Remembrance and connection to this sacramental seal brings quality and self-worth to the central plan of our life. The deep respect and integrity that we feel for ourselves and who we are, our Sacred Essence, in it's uniqueness as an expression of the Creative Force is what gives us our value. Our connection to our value allows for the expression of integrity in all our actions. Unblocking and activating this Energy Release Point connects us to our strong centre. A centre which is filled with vision born from knowing ourselves from True Self. Staying in our true alignment, we can express the gifts of our Divinity to fulfill our vision in its optimal expression and by so doing, live a purpose-filled life for the betterment of humanity.

Disharmonies: *Inability to find richness and fullness in life; lack of meaning to life; no identity; lack of self-confidence; low self-esteem; no pleasure in life; no pleasure in eating or receiving nourishment; indecision; inaction - the suspension of movement; paralysis; physical manifestations of cold in the legs; paralysis; pain in the genital region and disharmonies in the reproductive system.*

LIV-5 Insect Drain

Virtues: This Energy Release Point dispels annoyance over details by empowering a vision of the big picture. It focuses the mind inwardly toward our depths, restoring the nature of our Soul plan so that the mind can understand it. It brings empowerment of a deeper vision of the Divine Plan by helping to let go of attachments to specific outcomes. It clears the energetic field of negativity and toxicity of the environment as well as that brought on by psychic invasion. It enables the action of purification. The metaphorical significance of this Energy Release Point is that it depicts three insects. The number three corresponds in number to that of the three treasures or elixir fields that are cultivated through congruence of spirit, heart and vitality. These three treasures fuel our evolution and the emergence of all virtues during life. One must guard against the three insects who may drain or sap energy from our full body systems, by cultivating and strengthening these same treasures. The three insects are also the metaphor for illnesses that are attributed to evil spells cast by witches, as witches were believed to place many poisonous insects, worms and snakes in a container and to leave them there until only two were left. These final two were thought to reproduce and yield a toxin that could be transmitted to a person in order to afflict them. Unblocking and activating this Energy Release Point empowers the purification process necessary for the understanding of our Soul plan.

Disharmonies: *Frustration; aggravation; over-sensitivities to foods, chemicals and the environment; allergies; auto-immune disorders; excessive focus on details to the exclusion of the big picture; excessive attachment to our vision of how things should be, ought to be, or how they should look to others; judgement; resentment; fear; shame.*

LIV-6 The Metropolis / The Moon

Virtues: This Energy Release Point revitalizes and regenerates the whole body. It is appropriate that its name speaks to a place of great activity; a bustling centre where vitality of life is expressed. It is within this metropolis that one learns to navigate, spend and receive energy. The balanced use of giving and receiving energy. The Universal Principle of Compensation, within the Universal Principle of Cause and Effect. It is appropriate, therefore, to know how to guard and how to enhance one's life force through the quality of reciprocation and exchange, knowing that a cause will always have an effect and that experiences are a series of events. If one overextends energy there will be an effect. If one becomes energized through appropriate exchange, that too will create an effect. It is also appropriate that the alternate name for this Energy Release Point is the Moon. The Moon in many ancient traditions is venerated as a celestial body with magical, mystical and regenerative forces. The force of the Moon was seen as so great that it held great power over the Earth's waters - the waters in themselves a force of immense power. Ocean tides were co-related with the pull of the moon and had the ability to polarize the emotional body of humanity, as well as the animal and plant kingdoms. Several ancient cultures venerated the Moon for the attributes of mystery and miracles as well as for the elixirs of immortality and resurrection. (For example: Isis and Thoth in Ancient Egypt or Chenge in Ancient China who held the elixirs of immortality). Unblocking and activating this Energy Release Point empowers the energy of immortality, resurrection, revitalization and regeneration. Energy that is present within our cellular memories, that awaken to higher consciousness, allowing for a clear connection to the body's life giving forces.

Disharmonies: *Lack of motivation; loss of desire for life; weakness; devitalization; isolation; doormat syndrome; lack of involvement; inability to connect with vision, joy or life direction; inability to heal or recover from illness.*

LIV-7 The Flexible Network / Knee Pivot

Virtues: This Energy Release Point speaks to the virtue of flexibility. It is to be able to move in any direction, see life and respond to all angles. It strengthens the ability to see a vision, put a plan into motion and then to evaluate the plan midstream. Upon evaluation, the ability to see and make revisions is done with ease. Unblocking and activating this Energy Release Point creates a gateway for movement that has unlimited potential and possibilities.

Disharmonies: *Rigidity in mind and body; following the letter rather than the spirit of the law.*

LIV-8 Crooked Spring

Virtues: This Energy Release Point empowers the virtue of flexibility. It empowers the ability to flow around obstacles while staying focused on a goal, when the external context of our life conflicts with our plans. Strength and flexibility through two conditions. The first is through rootedness, which allows yielding without falling over. The second condition is emptiness, which represents non-attachment in the moment. After yielding to the temporary obstacle, one can spring up immediately to reassert purpose and resume the path. Unblocking and activating this Energy Release Point cultivates spiritual benevolence, brings suppleness and flexibility in thought and restores the quality of hope towards a brighter, happier and optimistic future.

Disharmonies: *Inflexibility and attachment to the outcome of plans and decisions; being at the point of "snapping" when minor stresses provoke anger; having a short fuse; compromise of our ideals in the face of challenges; despair; hopelessness; depression; inability to stand up for ourselves.*

LIV-9 Envelope of the Inner Feminine

Virtues: This Energy Release Point integrates feminine energy with human sexuality. It provides nourishment and nurturing to sexual activity through the honouring and respect of Self, thereby bringing sacredness to the physical act. For the Male, this Energy Release Point empowers the ability to sustain an erection. For the female, it nourishes the reproductive process for the co-creation and bearing of fruit. Unblocking and activating this Energy Release Point serves to integrate sexuality and spirituality into a sacred wholeness.

Disharmonies: *Resentment; polarization of sexuality and spirituality; sexual addiction; unfulfilled needs; sexual frustration; anger; physical manifestation of fibroids, endometriosis, cancer and inflammation of the prostate.*

LIV-10 Five Miles

Virtues: This Energy Release Point speaks to the Dynamic Law. It implies versatility, adaptation and activity in order to make progress. The physical location is on the leg, the appropriate anatomical part for movement. In ancient times, the Chinese symbol for this Energy Release Point was used to represent the length of the village road. Once one leaves the safety of the village and goes out into the world, the virtue of freedom and unexplored opportunities abound. Unblocking and activating this Energy Release Point renews the energy of excitement. It fuels the joyous realization that one can go anywhere and to do anything. It is the energy of freedom through adaptability and flexibility supporting the adventure of life experiences.

Disharmonies: *Fear; fear based spirituality which relies on religious ritual and sacrifice for salvation; overly influenced by the social expectations or values of family and/or community.*

LIV-11 The Feminine Angle of Modesty

Virtues: This Energy Release Point is a connection to the innermost recesses of the feminine energy, a place of privacy, hidden within each individual. Connecting with this Point allows for the flowing movement of stepping into our innermost desires, flowing action to our vision. It is to realize that which our Soul Blueprint has encoded into our physical structure. Unblocking and activating this Energy Release Point allows us to see into the beauty of who we are, in all of our mystery, as well as open our receptivity to embracing the softer inner self. Viewing that which was hidden, receiving guidance and the abilities to shape our life in order to live life to the fullest, all while empowering the virtues of modesty and humility. At the most profound level, Feminine Angle of Modesty empowers the process of re-birth after the period of darkness and shadow, achieving the highest level of creation.

Disharmonies: *Stagnation; stagnation due to victim consciousness; inability to see the beauty within; inability to recognize self-worth.*

LIV-12 Urgent Stirred Vessel / Goat Arrow

Virtues: This Energy Release Point embodies the energy of vital circulation for creativity. This creativity is directed towards pro-creation as well as fulfillment of life plans on all levels of the physical, emotional, mental and spiritual planes. It serves to harmonize the relationship between self-esteem and sexuality. This Energy Release Point strengthens the directional arrow, moving the vision of the soul and pointing it to the heart. In this directed place, one may take straightforward steps and actions in creative pursuits and life plans, or, one can express desire and sexuality as a pure force of love energy for oneself and in joyful union with another. As the name Goat Arrow, it refers to the Mythical God Pan, the faun - half man, half goat. Pan, the God of Nature, the wild and the shepherds. Pan is often associated with sexuality for he was known for his sexual powers, determination and endurance. Unblocking and activating this Energy Release Point unleashes wild, raw, vital creative energy. On the physical level, it enhances virility and endurance for the male and allows for surges of sexual freedom and the bliss of orgasm for the female. On the Emotional and Mental levels, unblocking and activating this Energy Release Point releases the fear of intimacy and allows for heart openings and positive vulnerability so that on the spiritual level, one experiences the blissful communion with the Divine, within a sacred union.

Disharmonies: *Misdirected sexual energy expressing as anger, frustration and sexual aggressiveness; envy; jealousy; low self-esteem; shame; violent sexual fantasies.*

LIV-13 Chapter Gate / Completion Gate

Virtues: This Energy Release Point is suggestive of being at the end of a transitory state - where all things complete, where one witnesses and acts upon the turning of a new leaf and moves forward into the next phase of life. Standing in the middle of the gate is not comfortable. From this Point one may choose to go backwards and dwell in the past, perhaps re-writing or re-cycling repetitive thoughts creating worry and stagnation. Or, one may choose to step towards new life experiences. Unblocking and activating this Energy Release Point dissolves walls that block vision and empowers the letting go of old injuries so that one may take the forward step and experience a healthy transition. It also unblocks creativity, allowing for free flow of written work and other artistic pursuits.

Disharmonies: *Frustration; stagnation; nostalgic holding onto the past; resentments; repetitive thought patterns; inability to form visions or goals; inability to keep things in perspective.*

LIV-14 Gate of Hope / Expectation's Door

Virtues: This Energy Release Point empowers hope and the quality of aspiration. We aspire to fulfill our purpose, and are inspired and drawn onward toward the highest potential in our life. Perceived obstacles are dissolved and we are empowered to find creative solutions with renewed optimism. To take action based on our commitments and goals. Being in the NOW. Living in the moment is considered to be very healthy, yet it does pose a fine balance - that of the inability to see into the future, yet to trust that all is going to proceed in a healthy, happy way. Within this element of trust there is balance, for it is the recognition and living co-creatively with the Creative Force. Through this co-creativity, clarity of vision is enhanced. When vision is clear, purpose becomes clearer. From this perspective one can allow for planning and foresight, as well as goal setting and achievement. All by being fully present in the NOW. The best decisions and plans therefore, are those which are harmonious and in alignment with one's purpose and Higher Self, thereby creating the feeling and appearance of free-flow, the virtues of ease and grace within manifestation of dreams and vision.

Disharmonies: *Hopelessness; mental torture; suicidal tendencies; apathy; internalized anger; melancholia; negativity and irritability; unrealistic* *expectations leading to disappointment; procrastination derived from the belief of having time in the future which prevents initiation of meaningful change.*

SECTION 4

Spiritual Portraits of the Energy
Release Points for the Extraordinary
Energy Release Channels

All of the Extraordinary Energy Release Channels have an opening and balancing Energy Release Point. It is through these Energy Release Points that the Extraordinary Energy Release Channel is activated. There are also Energy Release Points within the Extraordinary Energy Release Channel that may be blocked as well and may need attention.

Portraits of the Energy Release Points
for the Extraordinary Release Channel
of the Divine Feminine Matrix

Opening Point

LU-7 Broken Sequence

Virtues: This Energy Release Point empowers the function of receiving inner clarity and letting go; surrendering that which no longer serves. It speaks to the Universal Principle that All is Rhythm. We receive and let go. We take in and we move out; everything is rhythmic and everything has an ebb and flow. When we seek to control or stop the rhythm, the sequence or Divine order of things seems broken and chaos ensues.

Unblocking and activating this Energy Release Point activates a return to balance by strengthening clarity of the concept of detachment and finding centre.

Disharmonies: *Lack of clarity; feelings of loss and longing stemming from childhood; difficulty with letting go and moving forward. Physical imbalances can manifest as things interrupted or out of rhythm: menstrual cycles, sleep cycles, eating disorders.*

Balance Point

KID-6 Sea of Reflection and Illumination

Virtues: This Energy Release Point connects to the depths of the vast ocean of consciousness, the womb of creation, where the Divine Feminine births and generates the potentialities of the Soul. The sea is the Microcosm to the ocean and the individual is the Microcosm to the sea. The individual, therefore, is made of consciousness - as generated by the Divine Feminine and made active by the Divine Masculine. The oceans, seas, and water systems move and flow by this dynamic energy. The water itself is a reflection of both aspects of the Creative Force - for it holds depth and moisture of primordial being-ness and yet reflects light and activity of the sun, the moon and the stars as active expression of doing-ness. It is inner vitality of inner wisdom. Unblocking and activating this Energy Release Point creates the opportunity to witness the reflection of Soul self brilliance. A brilliance fuelled by illumination and wisdom. By connecting to this brilliance, the mind is illuminated to the unknown nature of Self, in all aspects - the gifts, the beauty, the fears; all that which is buried. It enables conscious connection, allowing reflection into wisdom and thereby healing and releasing that which hinders the full growth into a Self Realized Being.

Disharmonies: *Fear stemming from Karmic sources; shock; trauma; anxiety; feelings of urgency; easily overwhelmed by life circumstances.*

Channel Points

DFM-1 Meeting of the Inner Seas / The Golden Door / Ghost Store

Virtues: This Energy Release Point speaks to the great mystery of the conception of life itself. The miraculous moment when a sperm kisses the receptive egg and LIFE is born. Life born of the seeds of Essence of the Creative Force, transmitting on beams of LIGHT. Channelled through our parents, and therefore, connecting us into physicality and to the vastness of all our genetic lineage of past and potential future generations. Here is the place of Source, the waters, illuminated by Light consciousness, alchemically becoming a new temple to house the Soul. Here, there is a rich and vibrant energy. Unblocking and activating this Energy Release Point brings regeneration to the Spirit. Communication between the Soul and the Physical body is re-established so that vitality and strength are restored. As the name Golden Door implies, this Energy Release Point connects one to their source of preciousness, referring to the sacredness, wonderful awe of the mystery of embodiment. The breath and life as an incarnated Being. As Ghost Store, it is in reference to the deep mysteries of Resurrection. Mystery in itself meaning the unknowable. That which is concealed or kept hidden as all great mysteries are.

Disharmonies: *Inability to conceive: thoughts, ideas, projects or a child; barrenness; overwhelm; despondency; feeling as though one is drowning or in darkness; depression.*

DFM-2 Crooked Bone / Encircling Bone

Virtues: This Energy Release Point connects deep within the inner recesses of Being - a place of sanctity. It is to connect with whirling dynamic energy within a sacred enclosure; a spiral path to the deep mystique of the Divine Feminine. It is a place where many, through the misuse of sexual creative energy, have either sought to possess and draw from others in order to capture its power; or alternatively, use its power to ensnare, lure and capture the will of another. Energetically, this place holds the memories of our lives as well as the memories of the genetic lineage of the women and men from whom we have birthed. All life energy is channeled through this passageway. As the name Crooked Bone, this energy can hold the imprints of torture, oppression, discomfort, or the darkness of the enemy. As the name Encircling Bone, it is an energy of sanctity; that which brings forth the embryo of life and immortality, the innate creativity held within the packaged gift of life itself. Unblocking and activating this Energy Release Point allows access to transformation energy that serves to release that which is hidden in darkness and pain in order to uncover and retain the jewel. It allows for deep exploration of who we are, as well as protects and enhances the ability to create new life; to rebirth and to flow flexibly within the development of the structure of our inner purpose.

Disharmonies: *Impotence; powerlessness; feelings of oppression; humiliation; self deprecation; inferiority complex; submission; mental, emotional, physical and spiritual torture; manipulative tendencies; sexual addictions; fear; physical manifestations of disharmonies in the reproductive system.*

DFM-3 Central Pole of the Jade Spring

Virtues: This Energy Release Point brings a visualization of a central pole which connects the Earth to the Heavens via the physical body.

The Heavenly Point is known as the Central Polestar. The Polestar is an immovable fixed point in the heavens that in many traditions is used as a point of meditation. It is a point of calmness, balance and centre. The ancients viewed this Polestar as a central pole around which three other stars revolved - the depiction of the interaction of Heaven, Earth and Humanity. (The Three Treasures) It is from this balanced place that one can observe the flow of life and govern one's own ability to navigate all that presents during the journey. The walking of the path moves in a pure and sure-footed way. It allows for experiences of transformation, bringing moments of unlimited potential and growth. In this way, ultimate creativity can unfold and the treasured jewel can be birthed.

Disharmonies: *Exhaustion and fatigue; inability to stay grounded; inability to bring projects to fruition.*

DFM-4 Gate of the Source

Virtues: Visualize this Energy Release Point as the point in which one directly accesses the Divine Feminine Matrix - the raw power of the ocean source - the creation vortex of all Creative Forces - the portal of access to raw power at full throttle. The place where ALL is contained. This Energy Release Point is known by many names in as much as there are many names of the Creator - however, it is tapping into an energy even bigger than this. The womb of all creation and the gate of all life. The origin and source of the

Divine Feminine Matrix and as such, one of the three foundational builders of life to birth in physicality beyond the body, spirit and soul. From the ONE (Creative Force) births the TWO - the Divine Feminine Matrix and Divine Masculine Director - the Seeds of Life. This Energy Release Point is a sacred point used for anointing the physical body as it re-initiates it's affirmation to Life and Creation. Unblocking and activating this Energy Release Point connects us to the energy of the womb of creation.

Disharmonies: *Thoughts of anti-creation (suicide or murder); depletion; coldness; withdrawal; depression; inability to conceive (ideas, thoughts or a child); impotence; infertility; emaciation.*

DFM-5 Stone Gate

Virtues: This Energy Release Point connects with your main energy centre and carries a dual aspect. It can serve to unblock or block creativity, depending upon the intention of the individual and the use of free will. Ancient stone carries with it the consciousness of time through the wisdom of ages. It is solid yet smooth and holds great strength. A rock in itself is beauty in its stillness, and from the point of stillness one can examine and contemplate change, finding harmony within the imbalances that present through life experiences. Unblocking and activating this Energy Release Point with positive intention allows us to connect solidly to the centre of strength and wisdom. From this balanced place, one can evaluate life direction, pause and make plans, and find the vitality to flow through stagnation being empowered to live fully in the world.

Disharmonies: *Lack of energy; low vitality; lack of warmth; weakness; fatigue and stagnation in artistic and creative pursuits.*

DFM-6 Sea of Abundantly Flowing Energy

Virtues: This Energy Release Point speaks to the great fullness of vital life force energy which can be accessed through our conscious harmonizing of lifestyle patterns with the rhythmic cycles of nature. With this conscious connection, we experience more fully the subtleties of the flow of patterns of the sun and moon; the growth and decay of foliage; the seasons and the climates. This awareness draws to our full body systems the nourishment needed to restore the vitality we need to feed our passion for purpose and creativity, and by consequence, restore and strengthen our spirit. Unblocking and activating this Energy Release Point assists in the promotion of new ideas and the enhancement of creative pursuits by unleashing our vast potential. On the physical level, not only is vitality and well-being enhanced but the functions of fertility and reproduction are strengthened.

Disharmonies: *Low vitality; lack of enthusiasm; creative blocks; depression; infertility.*

DFM-7 Feminine Crossing

Virtues: The gift of the Divine Feminine Energy is that it invites us to go within for deep exploration of the spiritual, mental and emotional bodies. Through this exploration, we understand how the deep hidden components of who we are affect us physically. This Energy Release Point speaks to the exact place of intersection of these powerful energies - yet in a space which provides a place of stability, centre and anchor. It serves to unite, intertwine and integrate a solid core and brings harmony within the entire field of consciousness throughout our physical temple. Unblocking and activating this Energy Release Point connects us to the field of internal consciousness where strength can be generated for outward joyful action.

Disharmonies: *Depression; frustration; withdrawal; mental and emotional instability; suicidal tendencies.*

DFM - 8 Gate of the Watchtower of Spirit

Virtues: This Energy Release Point speaks to the life cord itself - the Spiritual cord. This is a strongly defended watchtower which speaks to forms of its power. The watchtower is home to the mystic, the superhuman, the Divine spark, the miraculous. Visualize the alchemical fire of the spark of spirit/soul essence kissing the physical consciousness and merging to create the spiritual/soul/physical being.....now visualize the time before this manifestation to the thought behind the physical creation in the Universal mind of the ALL. The creation of the pre-creation of life. Unblocking and activating this Energy Release Point strengthens the connection to The Eternal Source or Life cord.

Disharmonies: *Severe depletion without known physical cause; trauma; being worn down over a long period of time; resignation; encountering the Void within the Centre of Self with the inability to see Life.*

DFM-9 The Flowing Division of Water

Virtues: This Energy Release Point has a strong influence on fluids and all things related to fluidity, flexibility, balance, buoyancy, creativity, stagnation or pooling. Water can symbolically represent the primordial life of all things. Many times, energy consciousness or life force has been pictured as a "vast ocean" from which all life derives. Water has the beautiful quality of retaining it's essential energy no matter how many times it is divided. A droplet of rain therefore contains within it all essential elements of the wholeness from where it came. For ALL is in the ALL and the minutest part of the ALL contains ALL. This Energy Release Point represents the flowing division of water into the components of mind, body and spirit. It is a picture of water's ability to flow in all aspects, in all directions, and around obstacles, without losing it's wholeness as well as it's ability to keep it's balance. It is precisely it's ability to flow that it can be balanced and used to conform to any situation that presents. Unblocking and activating this Energy Release Point allows one to flow like water. It allows the access of the attributes of water and bring forward power and might, or it helps one remain in stillness and tranquility as the situation requires.

Disharmonies: *Rigidity; lack of clarity; stress leading to the creation of disasters; stagnation and creative blocks.*

DFM-10 Dark Gate Into the Core

Virtues: This Energy Release Point opens the gate into the depths of the core essence of Feminine Energy, a place of tranquility, profoundness and solitude. In this place, one can explore mysteries of the Self. It is the place which strips, releases and drains that which is no longer needed, leaving the raw, bare, essential self. The action of stripping bare is done easily, in a quiet tranquil manner. It is unassuming and unannounced. It is done in a sacred way - in One-ness - communing with the Divine. The old self dies, the new self is re-born through transformation. Unblocking and activating this Energy Release Point facilitates the process of letting go of the old in order to be able to transform and receive the new; to re-birth and grow in Evolutionary consciousness.

Disharmonies: *Inability to let go of the past; attachments to old grievances; over-identification and attachment with illusory parts of the Self; clutter and chaos in self and in the environment.*

DFM-11 Interior Strengthening / To Build Within

Virtues: This Energy Release Point addresses the ability to digest life in all of its aspects. The ability to release all that is extraneous and that which does not serve, to release the pain of grief and longing, as well as the griev-ances of the past in order to receive new inspiration. Unblocking and acti-vating this Energy Release Point empowers the flow of creative thought. It provides clarity and focus in the mind and connects more deeply with the ability to draw nourishment from the depths of the internal feminine source. The core of our Being is strengthened, our alignment with inten-tion is facilitated because the connection to intuition is enhanced. This Energy Release Point assists us in making a shift to a higher vibrational frequency while keeping ease in the body through harmony.

Disharmonies: *Indigestion; flu like symptoms; ascension sickness; anxiety; apprehension.*

DFM-12 Central Core

Virtues: This Energy Release Point speaks to the centre of nourishment where the strength of digestion brings vitality. As the centre, it can connect to the energy of the whole body systems including the sensory systems. With this vast network of connection it is vital to stay in balance, to rec-ognize and honour experiences that present and to allow for the rhythmic process of receiving and letting go. Unblocking and activating this Energy

Release Point keeps the calm and stability necessary for keeping on the path. It keeps one on centre, that is to keep the aim and to move straight to our target. It is only when off centre that difficulties can arise. From a place of strong centre, it is easier to digest life and move with what comes.

Disharmonies: *Worry; anxiety; indigestion; relationship problems showing up which affect the appetite, such as love sickness.*

DFM-13 Upper Heavenly Core

Virtues: This Energy Release Point empowers the ability to accept nourishment and nurturing. Nourishment has many sources. On the physical plane the Earth provides food. On the emotional/mental plane, nourishment comes through healthy relationships and support systems that help one move through life experiences. On the Spiritual plane one is nourished by inspiration. Inspiration to create, to brighten and to radiate our light. Unblocking and activating this Energy Release Point allows for a greater connection with the process of inspiration and nourishment from the Spiritual body. By so doing, wisdom and insight are brought forward and action ensues to bring harmony of nourishment to our full body system.

Disharmonies: *Rejection of nourishment and/or nurturing due to intergenerational patterns; physical symptoms of indigestion, heart pain and lack of appetite; emotional and mental imbalances such as love sickness and anxiety.*

DFM-14 Great Watch Tower

Virtues: This Energy Release Point connects us with our heart, our inner chamber where our sacred inner flame is kept. It is an important point to reconnect us with our passion, especially when our priorities start to become Ego centred as opposed to heart centred. Wanting to stand out in a crowd, seeking fortune, fame or recognition as opposed to serving with gratitude and humility. Universal Law dictates that when one connects to their Soul purpose and lives in service for the enrichment of humanity and the raising of consciousness, abundance will follow. Unblocking and activating this point assists in bringing forward our gifts in the energy of pure joy of heart expression - with a vigilance and dedication that is unattached to outcomes. This detachment allows for the flow of abundance to manifest as Universal Law intends it. This Energy Release Point also connects us to our inner wisdom and potential. It assists in strengthening our purity of intentions. Reconnection with our heart in this way further assists us to unify the mind, body and spirit so that when we put our hearts into what we do, our work flourishes with life, compassion and abundance.

Disharmonies: *Lack of passion; lack of enthusiasm; lack of motivation; emotional flatness; racing heart; addictions; mental confusion; lack of energy.*

DFM-15 Loving Protection of the Dove

Virtues: This Energy Release Point is the symbol of peace and love of the Holy Spirit. Unblocking and activating this Energy Release Point allows for the flow of Spirit to enter within. It creates comfort, peace and security. It is a welcoming of love, warmth and light. Love and self love in particular, is enhanced and this creates the strongest form of protection. It allows us to honour and respect ourselves and hold light. This ability to hold light becomes a great source of loving strength which radiates outwards from the wholeness of Being. It is through this wholeness of self and flow of the Holy Spirit that one can heal others through their presence of calm, peace and love.

Disharmonies: *Anxiety; disconnection from spirit; feelings of emptiness; low self worth; inability to give or receive love; co-dependence in relationships.*

DFM-16 Middle Palace Courtyard

Virtues: This Energy Release Point flows the sense of security, peace and protection of the Holy Spirit into the sacred palace of the Heart. It is the point which feels balance, harmony and centre through its alignment with the Soul Essence and the Centre Channel. It exemplifies our integrity and uprightness as we stand in wholeness of our nature, allowing inspiration to fill the Heart. The vibratory healing qualities of this Energy Release Point is to recapture a meditative tranquil state in order to experience deep peace, refreshment and regeneration. Unblocking and activating this Energy Release Point helps us to find ourselves and to receive inspiration from the point of centre so that we can reclaim our will in service to Divine Will.

Disharmonies: *Inability to find peace; inability to hold centre; difficulty navigating life as though overly influenced by the wills of the masses.*

DFM-17 Centre of the Inner Storehouse of Light

Virtues: This Energy Release Point accesses the palace of the Heart where the temple of Heaven is found. Within this temple, one moves deeper into one's spiritual potential and finds peace, joy and connection with cosmic love. It allows for the embracement of life with greater sensitivity to the needs of others and the Self. It strengthens the ability to Self Love. It brings tenderness to allow compassionate action from a place of safety and protection. Protection and safety because the temple of Heaven is within the centre of the storehouse of Light. Light of the I AM, Light of Essence, which is more powerful than any shadow. The Storehouse of Light is further guarded by the palace of the Heart. It is a place of sincerity, purity and illumination of wisdom. Unblocking and activating this Energy Release Point unveils the brilliance of the eternal threefold flame so that it may radiate and re-invigorate the entire body in order that one may fully experience the embodiment of love and be love. When one realizes that one is Love, one can manifest love in action in the performance of service to humanity from a place of devotion, seeing the divinity in all.

Disharmonies: *Inability to embrace life; feeling stuck; anxiety; difficulty navigating changes through transitional times; stifling emotions. Physical imbalances can include laboured breathing; asthma and other bronchial and lung conditions; difficulty swallowing food and receiving nourishment.*

DFM-18 Jade Hall / Precious Gem

Virtues: This Energy Release Point speaks to the purity and perfection of our Essence. It is the reconnection with the sacred temple where one's Essence was created and blessed. The place of home; heaven where the Divine Elixir of the God Force flows and solidifies into precious gems - the matrix for an individual's crystal structure and crystal core and Christ Consciousness grid. Unblocking and activating this Energy Release Point connects one to the virtues of humility, purity and correctness as well as to resonate and bring forward their individual soul note. A note, that when sung becomes a living expression of self. It emits a clear, full sound of beauty serving to amplify the light within. A light which allows one to see the beauty of radiance within, despite the harshness and scarring of earthly life experiences.

Disharmonies: *Feelings of inadequacy; low self worth; disbelief in our abilities; self-deprecation.*

DFM-19 Purple Palace

Virtues: This Energy Release Point expresses the sacredness of the physical body as the palace of the Soul. Purple is an imperial, majestic colour that is associated with dignity, royalty and spirituality. The Soul is sacred, the body is sacred, the energy body and the light body is sacred, as are the spaces through which the body moves. Purple Palace is also a reference to a heavenly pole star. Unblocking and activating this Energy Release Point opens the pathway of the heart chamber to the crown and extends it further to the Oversoul. Here, all abilities that the Soul has mastered and wants to bring forward in this lifetime can be accessed and mastered. Here is the place where we can access the Template of our Soul. It teaches us to create balance and harmony as conditions necessary to generate the ability to hold the Soul as sacred. Purple Palace teaches one to honour and respect the wisdom of the Soul. Through sacredness, we are better equipped to connect with the greatness of the ALL and embody our divinity.

Disharmonies: *Disconnection; self effacement; unexplained longing.*

DFM-20 Magnificent Floral Canopy

Virtues: This Energy Release Point connects our physical body to the beautiful Star Essence from whence our Soul birthed. Once this connection is re-established, the energy generated by the star can flow to us. These energies imbue in us the magnificence and beauty of star Light, as well as the qualities of the star. This energy is further integrated with the God-like virtues and qualities imbued in our makeup from the Creative Force within our physicality. Unblocking and activating this Energy Release Point allows for this flow of energy, an energy which enhances our Light and strengthen our whole body systems. From this enhancement of star Light, our energy field is strengthened. Feelings of shielding and protection bring us security so that we can breathe in fully the richness and beauty of life.

Disharmonies: *Addictions such as smoking or drugs which block living life to the fullest; physical manifestations can be asthma and other lung related conditions; insomnia.*

DFM-21 Jade Within the Pearl

Virtues: When one thinks of pearls we are reminded of treasure. A virtual treasure chest of Jewels of wisdom found through life experience. Jade Within The Pearl is wisdom, that has been cultivated to reveal the virtues of faith, humility and benevolent action to all living things. These virtues by nature empower purity. Purity of mind and body to be able to receive even more advanced wisdom from a place of sincere motivation and intention. The jade is the true treasure found within the pearl, the precious inner gem from which the virtues of goodness, humility, faith and radiance are magnified and righteousness aligns with World Service. This Energy Release Point assists in bringing realization of one's potential and devotion to one's purpose. Recognition of the difference between service and servitude. In addition, the ability to restore harmony and peace within oneself is enhanced through the ability to release negativity. Self confidence, self reliance, self sufficiency and well being is exponentially enhanced.

Disharmonies: *Indigestion of life; digestive disorders; barrenness; low self esteem; premature aging; narrow scope of vision; inability to see the bigger picture.*

DFM-22 Celestial Chimney, the Opening of the Heavens

Virtues: This Energy Release Point is located in the notch of the sternum at the base of the neck. It is a beautiful window or passageway that allows for the flowing movement of Spirit. It allows a connection between our body, which may feel heavy and oppressed, to the Universal Mind of the Creative Force. The passageway between Heaven and Earth. This Energy Release Point reminds us to evaluate our relationship to the masculine: our Solar aspects, our fathers, brothers and partners. It helps us to break through patterns of diminishment, severe mood changes, impetuous, unexpected self-destructive behaviours or situations. Celestial Chimney, The Opening of the Heavens is a conduit to the return to clarity from experiences of shock, fear or trauma. Unblocking and activating this Energy Release Point allows for a clear passage and facilitates the ability to express from the core of our Being. It strengthens the ability of clear thinking, reception of inspiration and enthusiasm. It reminds one to breathe and flow with the Universal breath. It empowers the dispersal of stagnation and forward movement through the realization that you may surrender to where you are in this present moment, even when in pain. Through the act of surrendering, pain is transmuted into forgiveness and release.

Disharmonies: *Asthma; bronchitis; sore and swollen throat; excess mucus and laboured breathing; inability to swallow food; oversensitivity to the remarks and observations of others; throwing up life; inability to accept life and life situations; stiffness of the tongue; inability to express; swelling of the back of the neck.*

DFM-23 Majesty's Spring

Virtues: This Energy Release Point speaks to the purity and vitality of a source of fresh spring water, bubbling up in confidence, freshness and clarity. This water springs forth from the Earth and carries within it's consciousness, the memories of knowledge, skills and talents derived from the experience of the journey. It empowers the view of perspective and the ability to look at life from all angles. This spring bursts through the Earth as a true embodiment of joy, humbled yet honoured to carry the consciousness of knowledge and wisdom. Unblocking and activating this Energy Release Point connects us to the Majesty's Spring source of purity, where we humbly recognize the brilliant sparkle of who we are and allow Light to shine into our crystal depths. It supports us to live our life and step into our majestic mastery so our ability to expand and share our knowledge, skills and talents with others is renewed with a freshness that gives our life meaning.

Disharmonies: *Constant seeker; thirsting for more due to our perceived inadequacies; lack of ideas; verbal dryness; loss of voice due to not wanting to be heard; lack of confidence; holding back our potential.*

DFM-24 Receiving Fluid

Virtues: This Energy Release Point is symbolic of raising our arms to receive throughout our physical body, the flow of Spirit in the form of heavenly ambrosia. Hence, it is purifying, washing and cleansing our mind, body and spirit. It is connecting to the Celestial Pool - the Vault of the Heavens. Unblocking and activating this Energy Release Point allows us to receive the fluids of Heaven in order to be cleansed of impurities and stagnation and thereby allowing for free flowing joy.

Disharmonies: *Stagnation; paralysis; releasing stifled grief and trauma.*

Portraits of the Energy Release Points for the Extraordinary Release Channel of the Divine Masculine Director

Opening Point

SI-3 Back Ravine

Virtues: This Energy Release Point brings the flexibility needed to overcome obstacles which block one from staying on their course. There are many paths to connection to soul purpose and vision, and regardless of which path we choose, the goal is to arrive at the final destination. Back Ravine brings flexibility to the process and assists in the navigation of life. It strengthens inter-dependence and clarity, allowing for the discernment to know how, and when, to ask for assistance in order to create situations of positive outcome. It strengthens trust in the Divine plan. Unblocking and activating this Energy Release Point empowers trust. A trust that comes from the connection to our inner wisdom and intuition. A trust that evolves from the practice of discernment and alignment to Truth. As one re-connects with Soul Purpose, the natural outcome is that the physical body benefits by being nourished from within. Back Ravine builds strong forces of vital energy, by generating the continual flow of trust when walking the path.

Disharmonies: *Lack of clarity; untapped forces of masculine forthrightness; lack of vitality.*

Balance Point

UB-62 Extended Vessel / Ghost Road

Virtues: This Energy Release Point assists in creating the space and containment required to receive, store and circulate higher wisdom and knowledge. It helps with discernment to see what is truth and how this truth is reflected in our life. To discern how we can weed out non-beneficial influences, release extraneous non-serving distractions and to retain the jewel of what is essential to the unfoldment of our life plan. The ability to receive and access Universal Truths and to consciously understand them becomes the blueprint and basis for beneficial co-creative action. Extended Vessel provides a container of resources so that we create a fulfilling life in which we not only develop our wisdom, but also transform our wisdom and Universal Truths through the extension of ourselves into the world by our acts of service to others. Unblocking and activating this Energy Release Point empowers receptivity and allows these wisdoms to flow into us and be held within stores of containment for use towards manifestation of an empowered life. In this way, we are facilitated to become conscious directors of life as well as express ourselves in service to others. As the name Ghost Road suggests, this Energy Release Point is a ghost point. It serves to release negative energies that disconnect one from inner truth, willpower and the directives of the Soul as well as blocking the ability to pay attention to the needs of the body.

Disharmonies: *Fatigue; depression; inflexibility; rigidity in the body; overstriving; inability to access clear focused thoughts. Physical manifestations of pain in the shoulders from over pushing and over work.*

DMD-1 Stairway to Heaven / Long and Strong Thrust of Energy

Virtues: This Energy Release Point has the role of providing strength and vitality to the entire spinal column of the physical body and to the entire Energy Release Channel of the Divine Masculine Director. The significance of this role is key to understanding that the Energy Release Channel of the Divine Masculine Director is one of the eight infinity vessels responsible for the manifestation of the physical body. This Energy Release Point reinforces and re-invigorates total vitality. The name Long and Strong Thrust of Energy refers to the penis, the point on the human body that a hard strike may cause paralysis or death. It is the point where the Divine Masculine Director unites with the Divine Feminine Matrix giving directive force to the ocean of potential energy - the manifestation of life. For the female body, it is connection to the vital, strong masculine energy, to feel powerful and vigorous, to excel, compete and emerge victorious. As the name Stairway to Heaven, this Energy Release Point represents the raising of vital creative energy. As this energy raises, there is alchemical purification of base animal reproductive instincts to higher levels of creator consciousness. Achieving spiritual union at the highest level. Vitality is replenished in the highest sense through the union of physical vitality and etheric vitality for overall complete renewal and reinvigoration. Unblocking and activating this Energy Release Point provides the vitality needed for emergence, manifestation, re-birth and creation.

Disharmonies: *Weakness; depletion; devitalization; lack of co-ordination; uncooperative body parts; feelings of distress and overwhelm; lack of drive.*

DMD-2 Loins Birth

Virtues: This Energy Release Point speaks to sexual desires. It is this Energy Release Point which seeks unification in order to transfer energy. It is a direct link to creative vital force energy and the necessary energy required for a sperm to fertilize an egg - the culmination of two becoming ONE and initiating the division of the cells, thus creating life. Unblocking and activating this Energy Release Point unleashes the vitality of excitement which fuels passion and desire to bring forward and direct the energy of creation. This creation is the energy of physical manifestation-whether it be a child or the driving force behind a masterpiece.

Disharmonies: *Impotence; experiencing a creative block; to stagnate; inability to manifest.*

DMD-3 Border of the Loins

Virtues: This Energy Release Point promotes flexibility in all aspects of Being - the physical, emotional, mental and spiritual bodies. In the physical structure it especially assists the lower back, leg and the knees. Border of the Loins helps keep both the feminine and masculine energies in balance. It is knowing when to assert and be pro-active as well as knowing when it is appropriate to step back and observe, reflect and receive inspiration for the next step. It is the positive collaboration of both dynamic energies so that one may walk through the passageway of life experience with a firmness of purpose, yet having flexibility within the plan.

Disharmonies: *Pain in the physical body, in particular the lower back and knees; feeling weak in the body; stagnation which can manifest physically as menstrual pain in women or prostate issues for men; the inability to move forward; numbness of emotions; not fully embracing life on earth.*

DMD-4 Gate of Life, Destiny and Purpose

Virtues: This Energy Release Point is the gate through which life steps forward into actualized manifestation. Conception of a child comes from the union of masculine and feminine vital forces. This gate is the door from which life emerges. It connects to primal raw power of the Cinnabar field: the reservoir of power and vitality. As a gate, it can open and close in order to adjust the energy flow in correspondence to what is required to accomplish the task at hand. The regulation of energy flow corresponds to the effectiveness with which the individual can align with purpose and destiny. In a purpose filled life that follows destiny, the energy supply is abundant and easily accessible. Likewise, when lower ego makes demands on the individual, there is a diversion from purpose, the gate closes and devitalization can occur. Unblocking and activating this Energy Release Point allows for the energy of the creative force to flow into the passage leading to the heart and ignite passion to fuel desire. It fuels the energy needed to fulfill the agreements based on the cosmic decree at our incarnation. Furthermore, this Energy Release Point allows for unification with purpose enabling the harmonious flow of life; a life that is enriched and renewed with vitality.

Disharmonies: *Devitalization; resignation; exhaustion; inability to rest; inability to recover physical vitality even after rest and relaxation.*

DMD-5 Suspended Pivot

Virtues: This Energy Release Point is a place of movement, transformation and change. It allows the Soul to express through the flow of Spirit. This Energy Release Point assists in balancing the nature of polarity which leads to indecision. It is to have clarity in decision making knowing that change is change, free of judgment of good or bad and that decision making is tempered with flexibility - allowing for more change. All experiences are opportunities for growth. Flexibility within change allows for the movement of energy, to flow unrestricted in the direction prompted by the Soul on the Path of Life. It assists in breaking through patterns of inaction created by anxiety and fear. Unblocking and activating this Energy Release Point allows for clear connection and alignment of Soul promptings enabling Spirit to flow movement energy with ease and trust.

Disharmonies: *Lack of certainty; lack of confidence in decision-making abilities; general anxiety; fear of change; anxiety around new situations and experiences; physical manifestations of pain in the mid and lower back; inability to twist at the waist.*

*If pain is excessive and debilitating, or if symptoms of Multiple Sclerosis, Parkinson's or other motor diseases are present, then there can be past lifetime memories held in the body of being tortured and/or executed.

DMD-6 Central Pillar

Virtues: This Energy Release Point promotes a strong central pillar - physically related to the strength of our spine. It is to be upright, so that one's inner strength, is in direct alignment with the decisive commitment to honour and respect one's Divinity and the I AM Presence. This renewed commitment to the Divine Will facilitates the Ascension process. The analogy is likened to Spirit as water flowing to the Ocean of the Soul and that the journey of elevated consciousness is being on a boat, whose strength and sturdiness is derived from one's integral centre and alignment to the Divine Will. Unblocking and activating this Energy Release

Point ensures that actions taken, are done from being in alignment with one's strong Central Pillar.

Disharmonies: *Lack of centre; lack of will; low self esteem or self aggrandizement and/or self righteousness; the inability to live or take a stand for one's beliefs or convictions; depression; physical pain in the spine where it feels as though one's back is "breaking in two".*

DMD-7 Balanced Central Pivot

Virtues: This Energy Release Point is a central pivot of vitality. Vitality which provides strength to versatile movement. It empowers the qualities of staying in centre and balance so that action can quickly accommodate and flexibly move through change. It is quick adaptation. As a pivot point it opens one to all possibilities and potentials to move gracefully into new directions and life experiences. Unblocking and activating this Energy Release Point keeps one grounded and centred while navigating the seen and unforeseen aspects of life. It keeps the body and mind flexible in order to discern appropriate action for the opportunities which present on the journey.

Disharmonies: *Disorganized action; confusing opportunities with distractions; physical manifestation of inflexibility; rigidity in the body and mind; narrow scope of vision; lower back pain; feelings of being stuck; indecision.*

DMD-8 Ease and Strength

Virtues: This Energy Release Point embraces the polarity of ease and strength. Ease bringing the state of comfort which is a feminine nurturing quality, and strength bringing a more masculine quality of firmness and power. This Energy Release Point serves to balance these two opposites by integrating masculine forthright, initiating power with the softer feminine comforting qualities. It is the ability to feel strong, yet be able to relax and release tension. Ease and Strength allows for flexibility in the physical body by circulating the feminine nurturing energy. Unblocking and activating this Energy Release Point allows for both the physical body and the etheric body to integrate more easily and harmonize more effectively. In this way, new experiences are greeted with joyous grace and ease.

Disharmonies: *Emotionally, mentally and spiritually feeling smaller than you are; stiffness in the physical body; muscle tension; pain and inflexibility; inability to embrace life; feeling caged; insecure; overwhelm; ungrounded; walking aimlessly about.*

DMD-9 To Reach the Utmost High

Virtues: This Energy Release Point is the embodiment of moving from a place of sorrow and darkness, to transcend and bring about a resurgence of energy and vitality. It is a point which brings one to the visualization of heaven and the sensory cognition of the fifth dimensional vibrational frequency. It further allows one to re-connect to the Ultimate potential of one's Essence as birthed by the Creative Force. To Reach the Utmost High brings these potentials to fruition and manifestation into physicality. Unblocking and activating this Energy Release Point helps bring about re-alignment with integrity and strength while accessing inner fortitude to continue.

Disharmonies: *Depression; lack of vision; fatigue.*

DMD-10 Supernatural Tower / Spirit Tower / Spirit's Platform

Virtues: This Energy Release Point speaks to the connection with Spirit and our psychic openings. It is to be vigilant and observing of psychic phenomena and keep it in balance with the Heart Centre. That is to release fear, fanaticism, sensationalism and exaggeration. Unblocking and activating this Energy Release Point assists one to be aware of subtle sheaths which separate the dimensions of the material world - our physicality, from the lower and higher astral world of the fourth and fifth dimensions. The Virtues of vigilance is refined and the distinction between benevolent and malevolent Beings are at a heightened awareness, thus allowing for higher choices of connection to Forces of Light to predominate. As one allows for more Light to enter the consciousness, one can more easily shift perspectives from a material view of life to one based on sacredness of the heart.

Disharmonies: *Fear; obsessive thoughts; preoccupation with death and things of a macabre nature; confusion and the inability to think clearly; physical ailments such as asthma, bronchitis and coughs.*

DMD-11 Spirit Path

Virtues: This Energy Release Point calms the spirit, the mind and the body. It is when the mind is quiet that one can hear the gentle whispering of the Soul. Spirit Path frees the thinking mind and helps find mental repose and inner peace. It brings a calm and centred energy so that one can create the space to evaluate life direction. As the mind calms, the Heart's wisdom calms the fear in the body. Unblocking and activating this Energy Release Point calms the mind and body so that one may perceive Soul purpose, find courage and strength, and thereby create an environment for a gentle unfoldment of Life's path.

Disharmonies: *Chattering mind, indecision, fear of change, obsessive thinking.*

DMD-12 Sustaining Pillar of Life

Virtues: This Energy Release Point strengthens the spine and assists in rejuvenation and regeneration of the full body system. This pillar is a column of support; one which stays erect and tall as well as sustains existence. Rooted deeply into the Earth, yet suspended by Heaven, it allows one to connect with the inner strength of integrity. It builds courage and backbone to stand up for one's truth, as well as strengthens the ability to go on. Unblocking and activating this Energy Release Point strengthens ones inner structure. With this structure, life can grow and flourish. A structure which generates and sustains a renewing, creative and nurturing cycle. As one learns to ground in their Essence, one becomes more fully rooted and the ability to draw nourishment and sustaining energy from the Earth, as well as the ability to receive more heavenly inspiration is amplified.

Disharmonies: *Stress; the appearance of everything crumbling around you; uprootedness; isolation; inability to stay in centre and fully in the body; inability to find one's place on Earth.*

DMD-13 Kiln Path / Fires of Transformation

Virtues: Kiln Path/Fires of Transformation is also known as the Road to Happiness. In the name Kiln Path, the kiln in this circumstance refers to the ceramic amulets of the Taoists, who wore these to ward off evil spirits. The Ancients knew that clay shapes worn as amulets would assist in keeping one on the true path by protecting from the external influences designed to lead astray. With the higher vibrational energies entering and now present on the larger planetary system, earth alchemy is also presenting humanity with crystal amulets - crystal consciousness to protect our evolution and to connect us to the crystalline grid and transformative energy of our time. This Energy Release Point also speaks to the fire of alchemy and transformation. It is the place where aspects and parts combine in order to birth a Great Creation. This creation is then given a form, a time and a space. This form is fuelled by passion, love and beauty, and consequently it transforms yet again into something of endurance - perpetuity. It is here that one may grasp the concept and fully understand what it is to be immortal. It is to know that our lifestream is eternal and by connecting with the ALL we can choose a true path; one that flourishes and is filled with joy. Unblocking and activating this Energy Release Point brings connection to transformational fires. It activates a protective energy, an etheric amulet which serves to keep one safe on the path, strongly protected from distractions of the dark.

Disharmonies: *Prone to parasitic influences; entity invasion; disrespect for life; blunted feelings; disconnection from Source; over-attachment to temporal personality; fear of death.*

DMD-14 Great Hammer / Hundred Taxations

Virtues: This Energy Release Point is symbolic of a cosmic hammer that has the ability to prompt great change by bringing forth the energy of movement. It is particularly effective when one has overtaxed the physical body with hard labour; emotional distress or mental exhaustion and fatigue from over striving. This Energy Release Point serves to bring up great reservoirs of energy to release burdens, relieve pain in the physical body and calm the mind. It brings one to great awareness that lifestyle changes are necessary in order for the spiritual body to integrate with more ease with the mental, emotional and physical bodies. Once this awareness is brought into consciousness, the spiritual body can flow with healing grace. Unblocking and activating this Energy Release Point unleashes dynamic energy that provides release of painful imbalances, as well as quickens the re-integration of the spiritual body, so that soul inspiration for positive forward movement is more ably received.

Disharmonies: *Physical body pain; stress; disorders in the lung due to the stagnation of inspiration; discouragement; inability to move the neck in order to see from a higher or different perspective.*

DMD-15 Gate of Dumbness / Loss of Voice

Virtues: This Energy Release Point expresses the metaphorical place of juncture, that is to reach a turning point. It is precisely at this place where the key is found to unlock the gate of vocal repression. Unlocking and walking through this gate empowers the ability to speak the necessary words to bring to a resolution an inner conflict, or the experience of a present reality, that is not in alignment with the inner self. Unblocking and activating this Energy Release Point opens the gate that fear or insecurity locked shut. It enables one to be able to speak, to sing and to laugh in freedom, thereby bringing healing in right relationship within Self and with others.

Disharmonies: *Repression leading to loss of voice; loss of self empowerment; loss of higher creativity; there can be bitterness, distaste or dislike of a situation; a loathing, or to tire of a situation leading to mis-use of the spoken word; physically there can be an affliction of the tongue or throat.*

DMD-16 Palace of the Wind / Ghost Forest

Virtues: This Energy Release Point speaks to the wind and the changes that the wind brings as well as the effects of atmosphere and vibration on one's physical, emotional, mental and spiritual state. It allows for the observation and awareness of the outside environment, (chaos, change, temperaments, astrological influences and planetary change for example) yet staying in a detached larger perspective so that one does not become embroiled with the waves of mass fear or hysteria that tumultuous times can bring. This Energy Release Point is susceptible to exterior influences and viewed somewhat like a gate, or doorway to the palace: the home of your divinity. This passage therefore must be on guard to exterior influences and entity intrusion for it is here that thought forms or entities enter. In physical reality, it is known that a blow to this point will most likely result in physical death. In emotional, mental and spiritual realities a psychic blow to this point will most likely lead to a fracturing and possible mental/emotional illness or energetic death to a soul aspect or part. Unblocking and activating Palace of the Wind/Ghost Forest brings awareness and a renewal of vitality to strengthen and energize the whole body system, creating a heightened response for increased self defence.

Disharmonies: *Weakened immune system; obsessive thoughts; low vitality; over sensitivity to the external environment; susceptible to mass hysteria and anxiety; easily influenced by group thought.*

DMD-17 Brain Door / Brain Household / Encompassing Wind

Virtues: This Energy Release Point speaks to the entryway of the brain, our thoughts, realizations, practices, manner, deportment, skills and comprehension. All brain function on many levels, from the unconscious abilities of body regulatory functions to higher thought processes and beyond. This doorway serves as a connection from the brain to the heart. Unblocking and activating this Energy Release Point allows for the brain to be directed from the heart - to be governed by the passion, understanding and intuitions of the heart. Insight and wisdom guide our thoughts, words and actions, and decisions can be made from balanced reason.

Disharmonies: *Unclear communication; mental agitation; lack of focus; easily distracted; subject to invasive energy which can cause the physical manifestation of epilepsy.*

DMD-18 Strength Between / Great Feather

Virtues: This Energy Release Point has the physical location of being part of the sacred geometry in the back, which forms a triangular shape. This shape is much like that of an archer's bow. It's location within this triangle is the centre, hence it's name: The Strength Between two halves. The strength between comes from being in centre and balance - for this is the Universal Principle of Power. Here one can connect and reflect on inner wisdom and become the master of one's life. This can also be likened metaphorically to the moon as seen through a window, a moon framed by the curtains on each side. The moon as an illuminator, shining through these halves draws us inwards to contemplate and reflect on the messages found within. The alternate name: Great Feather, speaks to the archer's arrow, flying straight and true to it's ultimate goal. It is unyielding, focused and strong. It's energy directed toward the fulfillment of purpose as aligned with Soul Essence and as directed by the Higher Self. The aim is clear and accurate. Unblocking and activating this Energy Release Point brings strength from a place of centre and balance so that one can stand in self empowerment and respond in action for the benefit of highest good of self and for the benefit of ALL.

Disharmonies: *Loss of internal vision, purpose and direction; withdrawal and isolation; inflexibility; emotionally and physically one may be experiencing depression and insomnia.*

DMD-19 Posterior Summit / Behind the Vertex

Virtues: This Energy Release Point speaks to an intersection point where groups, ideas or events meet. As a point of intersection, there can be chaos and clashing confusion. This Energy Release Point connects to energy which serves to harmonize consciousness so that there can be flexibility and receptivity. Unblocking and activating this Energy Release Point allows for the expression of emotion so that discordant energy can be diffused. It promotes clear communication which is emotionally balanced so that ideas can be nourished. It promotes strategy for harmonious living, enriching feelings of contentment that one has spoken, has been listened to, and is now calm. In this state, life goals and plans can forge ahead in a renewed harmonious state and the sense of peace and order is restored.

Disharmonies: *Anger; discontent; stagnation and withdrawal; feelings of imminent crisis and fracture.*

DMD-20 Meeting in Grand Unity / One Hundred Convergences / The One, Three and Five

Virtues: This Energy Release Point embodies the Hermetic axiom "As Above, So Below". It is the meeting place of unity with the Creative Force. It is the point of unification where the Creative Force interfaces with the physical body through the seventh energy centre and into the centre channel. It is the reflection that all that is contained in the Cosmos, the Macrocosm, is contained within the individual, the Microcosm. It is where everything from a place of wholeness is directed into the One. Unblocking and activating this Energy Release Point unleashes a flow of vitality born of creativity and inspiration, serving to energize the full body systems. It serves to reconnect to ancient wisdom from both the spiritual and genetic lineages in order to bring our individual lifestreams into harmony. It restores balance, tranquility and calm. This flow of energy continues to serve the energetic system of the body through its connection to the seventh energy centre, and from there to the other energy centres, sensory and secondary centres, the central, main and core channels, the

Energy Release Channels, the Energy Body and the vertical and horizontal fields. It is through this Energy Release Point and it's flow of continual energy that magnetizes the effects of prayer, new belief systems and meditation. In addition, this Energy Release Point has the numbers one, three and five connected with it. This is seen as the movement created through the intervals of music in the pentatonic scale. (The basic scale in Chinese culture) Music is a universal language spanning all cultures and ages. The movement of thirds embody movement within movement itself, therefore speaking to the swiftness and enormity of the movement of spirit and manifestation. The One represents the energy of the ALL descending into physicality, creating the blueprint of an individual life stream. The Three becomes the manifestation of physicality through union of the masculine and feminine energies creating the Being. The Five is representative of the Being in a perfected state, the embodiment of a Divine Soul animated by Spirit.

Disharmonies: *Feeling of fragmentation, fragility and overwhelm; weakness; depletion; disconnection from spirit, from purpose, from life; anxiety.*

DMD-21 Heavenly Anterior Summit

Virtues: This Energy Release Point is the place in the heavens where meetings are held. Heavenly Anterior Summit has a dual meaning. Summit being a point that is higher in elevation than all points immediately adjacent to it; summit being a meeting of heads of state and the common expression for global governance. When these two meanings are integrated, this becomes a place of connection to Higher Self, a raising to a higher vibrational consciousness. To connect with this summit allows for harmonization, an opportunity to diffuse a potential crisis, event or chaos, while still having an opportunity to affect and make changes to circumstances. Hence this empowers the conscious co-creator. It is connecting with the function of the Divine Masculine Director in that it oversees or governs the purposeful activity of the individual lifestream's journey through life. Unblocking and activating this Energy Release Point brings us to the place of clarity and wisdom through conscious connection to the

Higher Soul Aspect. It strengthens and stabilizes Spirit and expands our vision in regards to life direction by connecting to the wholeness of the ALL.

Disharmonies: *Lack of clarity; chaos; inability to focus and be in present time; instability through times of shifting; distortions in perception of reality. Physically this calms epilepsy, dizziness and vertigo.*

DMD-22 Skull Meeting / Ghost Gate

Virtues: This Energy Release Point is likened to a skylight. A place where the light enters through the crown of the head and streams forth to the heart. This streaming light energy therefore brings communication via light from the Heavens to the deep recesses of the heart. The heart in return releases energy that fed the ghosts of sorrow, isolation and with-held pain through the flowing of tears, of sighs or of laughter. Musically it represents the third tone - the third in itself is an interval which holds the energy of movement or a flow - a gateway or passage way - bringing with it under-standing, comprehension and realization. Further aspects of the third is the exploration of the triplex bond of unity: Divine Masculine/Divine Feminine and wholeness of Body; Father/Mother/Child; Body/Spirit/Soul for a few examples. Unblocking and activating this Energy Release Point brings heightened awareness to full Soul expression. An expression which moves one to evolve, develop, grow and unfold, ultimately leading to the perfected manifestation of Being.

Disharmonies: *Mental fatigue; stifled creativity; inability to experience mind/heart connection; inability to work cooperatively with others; physical manifestations of headaches and dizziness.*

DMD-23 Heavenly Star / Spirit Hall / Ghost Mansion

Virtues: This Energy Release Point draws it's vibrancy and name from the interaction of three heavenly stars. The interaction of these three heav-enly stars become the metaphor of the generation of life. It is a point of creation, ascension and transformation - the endless cycle of resurrection and life. These are the points of light through which Spirit vibrates, creating our individual Soul note. It is spontaneous creative power. As the name Spirit Hall, this Energy Release Point invokes connection to Spirit in the purest sense. As Ghost Mansion, one becomes aware of the treasured sacredness of our individual life stream and purpose. This is a sacredness which one must guard, honour, respect and protect. Unblocking and activating this Energy Release Point brings connection. Connection to an inner vision which beholds the path of illuminated cosmic wisdom and the Soul's plan for the individual life stream within the Universal tapestry towards Ascension.

Disharmonies: *The inability to see; the inability to think for oneself; disconnection from purpose, from Source, from life; living a shadow of one's potential; experiencing emptiness and hollow existence due to entity invasion and parasitic influence.*

DMD-24 Sacred Courtyard of the I AM

Virtues: This Energy Release Point allows one to see and recognize the Divine in all things. Not only in the Beings that surround us, but to be able to see and recognize the Consciousness of the Divine in all the kingdoms. The mineral, plant and animal, as well as the consciousness behind, within and manifest in the experiences of living. Activation of this Energy Release Point unlocks the space of vibration to the inner chamber of wisdom - a sacred place through which one connects to the qualities of quiet contemplation and tranquility. It creates a space within this place that has a goal and intention to prepare one to meet with the ALL or God Force. It further enhances the understanding that to remain present, in the Now moment, amplifies the ability to see the Creative Force in action. Everything that presents in form of observation and experience brings understanding through spiritual revelation. Unblocking and activating this Energy Release Point empowers spiritual enlightenment through the suspension of time. It is an Energy Release Point of Illumination.

Disharmonies: *Feeling lost or having strayed from the path; anxiety; head-aches; difficulty finding rest and comfort; no sense of where is home; mental turmoil; mental disorders; psychosis and schizophrenia.*

DMD-24.5 Hall of Impression / Seal Hall

Virtues: This Energy Release Point is the place from where our I AM presence and purpose shine. The place which streams forth Light and connects our Divinity to the ALL. It is the place where we see ourselves as we truly are. It is our sacred identity and not Ego based. It is associated with the Creative Force, the movement of Spirit, the Primal Source. It is associated with the Heart, not the personality. It is Conscious Spirit. This Energy Release Point is also the 13th ghost point which exists on the physical body, meaning that it is a place where there is the vulnerability of allowing energy in that serves to block us from seeing who we truly are. Unblocking and activating this Energy Release Point empowers a true vision of who we are and why we are here, thereby allowing for Divine connection to our gifts and living the full expression of our potential.

Disharmonies: *Not seeing ourselves as we truly are through our own eyes; seeing ourselves through the eyes of another and picking up their perceptions of reality, creating issues of judgment and lack of esteem.*

DMD-25 The Simplicity of the White Unadorned Bone

Virtues: This Energy Release Point allows one to return to the place in consciousness of the bare Essential Self. The simplicity, the bare bones, the basic structure of who we are. Bones are the foundation, they are strong and house the marrow, which in turn regenerates the cells of our body. It is through the bones that our body can transform. Bones holds the memories of life and continue to do so long after the time of transition of a Being or an animal. The reference to white is the reference to purity and simplicity, such as the purity of a white silk thread which creates the cocoon of the silkworm. This purity sets the condition or environment for transformation and rebirth. This simplicity speaks to all aspects of life:

food, material possessions and lifestyle. Returning to Simple Abundance and by so doing, unlocking the Secret of the Golden Flower; the origin of a new Being in the place of power. Unblocking and activating this Energy Release Point brings one to the cocoon. A place of transformation in which one sits, breathes and contemplates the becoming of the Golden Flower.

Disharmonies: *Dissatisfaction; chaotic life; inability to find peace or tranquility.*

DMD-26 Waterway to the Centre of my Being / Ghost Guest Room

Virtues: This Energy Release Point speaks to the importance of placing oneself first in order to be able to assist others. This Energy Release Point has as a main function the empowerment of resurrection and resuscitation - to bring back the Essence when disconnection from both the energies of the Creative Force and the Earth Mother have parted company. When there is a disconnection from Essence (Creative Force) and vital life forces (Earth) the Being in the physical body is in a vulnerable state. It is in this vulnerable state that mental/emotional and physical fracturing can occur. Fracturing to the extent of becoming a host to astral entities, dark forces and fear based thought forms as the alternate name Ghost Guest Room suggests. Unblocking and activating this Energy Release Point allows for the flow of harmony from Divine Sources to reach the core of our Being. It is through the connection to the inner core that wisdom reigns. When wisdom is established, purpose and direction finds the Path. Once on the Path, one can resume the walk through life in simplicity, cultivating peace, harmony and joy.

Disharmonies: *Devitalization; exhaustion and fatigue; fear; poverty and survival consciousness; entity invasion; obsessive thoughts.*

DMD-27 Correct Exchange / To Open With Correct Reason and Happiness

Virtues: This Energy Release Point empowers us to open up and exchange through the spoken word, the truths of our right alignment. As we go through life, we are often met with a diversity of experiences that help define our internal measure of what becomes our truth. Here, at this Energy Release Point, we are open to experiencing opportunities which present to us in the NOW moment. These opportunities and our words, are made manifest and should we choose, we can be propelled more and more forward towards a purpose filled life. Subsequently, the more in alignment we choose to become, the more clarity we gain. All becomes clear and synchronistic. Unblocking and activating this Energy Release Point helps us speak intentional words. Words that create actions which become more and more in alignment with our Divine Self, thereby bringing joy and happiness in all aspects of Being.

Disharmonies: *Withdrawal; congestion; indecision; clenched jaws; rigidity.*

DMD-28 Mouth of the River Crossing Into the Sea

Virtues: This Energy Release Point speaks to the ending and the beginning. The end of a passage, a chapter or a cycle in life and the beginning of a new creation. To become, to explore or to move into. It is to be able to extract value and accumulated wisdom from the experience of living and bring these qualities of value and wisdom forward into the creation cycle. With all life, the Universal Principle of Rhythm engages in an endless cycle of movement and transformation Unblocking and activating this Energy Release Point strengthens the alchemy of flow within the Wholeness of the ALL. An alchemy which harmonizes the mind, the body and the spirit through breath and movement with the Universal pulse.

Disharmonies: *Needing to be in control; inflexibility; fear of change; stagnation.*

Portraits of the Energy Release Points for the Extraordinary Release Channel of the Penetrating Interface

Opening Point

SP- 4 Yellow Emperor / Grandparent-Grandchild

Virtues: This Energy Release Point is the only Energy Release Point on the body with a royal name. It speaks to human history that is found in mythology. In this mythology one finds a distant Divine ancestor representing Heaven, as well as a distant ancestor representing Earth. In this respect it serves to unify the light of the Mind of Heaven with the passion of the Heart of Earth. It is to be unselfish, to be open to all and to create and share posterity for the benefit of humanity. This Energy Release Point also is the family name of the mythological Yellow Emperor who ruled China for 100 years from 2697 BC to 2597 BC. It is symbolic of gold, royalty, merit, youth, virginity, happiness and fertility. It is the Yellow Emperor that received ancient wisdom of medicine to help ease the suffering of his people. He taught them to be stewards of the Earth and the Earth in turn would nourish the nation. By tending the Earth and teaching future generations the ability to do the same, the Emperor could be assured that prosperity, stability and abundance would be the birthright of all the descendants of his people. In this way, future generations would continually reap the riches of the harvests and as such this would be the inheritance of the royal treasury. Unblocking and activating this Energy Release Point empowers the unification of generations. It forms a bridge between the wisdom of the past and brings hope for the future. It unites and strengthens the ability to act in accordance to the heart's passion while strengthening the forces of will. Yellow Emperor combines strength with wisdom and creates hope and optimism for the future generations in order for humanity to continue the journey.

Disharmonies: *Dysfunctional comfort seeking behaviour; addictions or addictive behaviour; being disheartened and depressed; hopelessness; pessimism and despair; conflict with images of authority; alienation from the past; disconnection with genetic lineage; unconscious wasteful behaviour* *in regards to environmental issues; disconnection from nature; unconscious exploitative behaviours in regards to nature.*

Balance Point

P-6 Inner Frontier Gate / Inner Palace Gate

Virtues: This Energy Release Point embodies our journey into our hearts - the frontier and unexplored territory known as the borderlands. The journey into this transition zone cannot help but create transformation - for in the act of undertaking the journey itself one is transformed through the encounter of the unknown. As a gate point, one is empowered to come and go at will understanding the appropriate boundaries in relation to the sanctity of the Heart and sharing oneself with others. Qualities of compassion, connection, warmth and light are accessed and bring the perseverance to proceed onward with the journey. Unlocking the gate to this inner heart space signifies a profound turning point for the one willing to pass through and transform pain and hurt into blessings of peace and calmness. Unblocking and activating this Energy Release Point can assist in calming the Self from the trauma of betrayal from intimacy, rape, incest or divorce.

Disharmonies: *Closing the heart in self protection from the pain of intimacy; projecting old pain onto the present; feelings of being stabbed or shot in the heart due to betrayal or painful separations.*

Crossing Points

DFM-1 Meeting of the Inner Seas / The Golden Door / Ghost Store

Virtues: This Energy Release Point speaks to the great mystery of the conception of life itself. The miraculous moment when a sperm kisses the receptive egg and LIFE is born. Life born of the seeds of Essence of the

Creative Force, transmitting on beams of LIGHT. Channelled through our parents, and therefore, connecting us into physicality and to the vastness of all our genetic lineage of past and potential future generations. Here is the place of Source, the waters, illuminated by Light consciousness, alchemically becoming a new temple to house the Soul. Here, there is a rich and vibrant energy. Unblocking and activating this Energy Release Point brings regeneration to the Spirit. Communication between the Soul and the Physical body is re-established so that vitality and strength are restored. As the name Golden Door implies, this Energy Release Point connects one to their source of preciousness, referring to the sacredness, wonderful awe of the mystery of embodiment. The breath and life as an incarnated Being. As Ghost Store, it is in reference to the deep mysteries of Resurrection. Mystery in itself meaning the unknowable. That which is concealed or kept hidden as all great mysteries are.

Disharmonies: *Inability to conceive: thoughts, ideas, projects or a child; barrenness; overwhelm; despondency; feeling as though one is drowning or in darkness; depression.*

ST-30 Rushing Energy / Thoroughfare of Energy

Virtues: This Energy Release Point has the ability to harmonize energy that has a tendency to rise up with sudden swiftness. It is a modulator or balancer which calms the rush and allows for a smooth flow of energy that brings nourishment to the heart and calmness to the mind. Within this process, this Energy Release Point clears the pathway from the heart to the mind, allowing free flow through the neck, where panic energy can gather and re-route it to where it belongs - in the third energy centre. The empowerment of the third energy centre allows for clearly directed will forces. By conscious connection to the will, one can then restore their authentic power, a power which releases control, manipulation or passivity when in relationship with others. Unblocking and activating this Energy Release Point harmonizes energy to empower life. It calms the emotional body and balances any feeling that produces agitation. It promotes self care which integrates nurturance, as well as nourishment received from positive life experiences. It helps one to trust in the smooth unfolding of life's path. It assists in the ability to open emotionally and form deep committed intimate relationships, as well as facilitates the integration of spiritual life forces within the physical being.

Disharmonies: *Overwhelm; fear; fear of exposure; vulnerability; intimacy issues; panic; anxiety; suppressed sexuality; feelings of isolation and separation; digestive disorders leading to acid reflux; heart palpitations; hot flashes; gynaecological disorders; lower abdominal pain; impotence; hunger with no desire to eat.*

KID-11 Horizontal Bone / Curved Valley

Virtues: This Energy Release Point connects to the deepest recesses of our Essence through the marrow of our bones; a place where we will never be shaken or thrown off for it is the absolute core of who we are. In reaching this place, we can cleanse and transform ourselves through the vitality likened to that of a seed bursting into life holding the inherited pattern of our potential. Here is the inner core of strength, which serves to hold our integrity while protecting our Essence. This Energy Release Point also assists with the integration of our spirituality with our physical sexual function honouring the sacred wholeness. Through conscious unity, the sexual act becomes sacred. The conception and incubation of life is likewise a sacred service of Divine love. Unblocking and activating this Energy Release point allows for the reception of Divine inspiration, enhancing the ability to bring all creative projects to fruition.

Disharmonies: *Inner torment and Hell; self destructive tendencies; suicidal thoughts; self mutilation; feelings of oppression; being enmeshed in situations of dilemma and predicaments; shame and fear associated with sexuality and sexually transmitted diseases; feelings of impotence; lack of creativity; feelings of aloneness and experiencing the valley of the shadows; feeling that life keeps throwing curves and twists on the path; polarization of sexuality and spirituality; sexual addictions.*

KID-12 Great Glorious Brightness

Virtues: This Energy Release Point empowers conception - the conception of ideas or the conception of a child. It stimulates the sexual energy centre, also known as the creativity centre, to enhance creativity and empower growth. It is the sun and it's glorious bright solar energy that, with it's warmth, allows for the growth and flowering of plants. It is also the full engagement of feminine earth energies with the masculine solar power that create the ideal environment for life and growth to flourish. Likewise, in our intimate sexual relationships, full engagement of the sexual energies in the body with that of spiritualized energy of the Divine Masculine and Feminine forces will lead to glorious fulfillment and bliss of a sacred union. Unblocking and activating this Energy Release Point allows the solar aspects of healthy Ego strength to illuminate the feminine depths within, promoting our ability to transcend fear and shame. It is the balanced Ego strength that allows the transformation of fear into wisdom of the Heart. When this transformation happens, the Heart unwraps itself to open, receive and share it's depths of love and authenticity with positive vulnerability. Introspection and healing warmth are activated as the Heart opens to the warmth of trust. Thus commences the process of a compassionate cleansing of the subconscious of the shadow, along with integrating spirituality with sexuality.

Disharmonies: *Fear of intimacy; fear of the unknown; excessive blushing; shyness; lack of confidence; shame in regards to sexuality; coldness and frigidity; inability to relax; problems with conception.*

KID-13 Door of Infants

Virtues: This Energy Release Point opens, nourishes and encourages vital bursting of energy. It is this energy that is present and shows strength in the birthing of a baby, the blossoming of a flower and in the hatching of an egg. It is an energy that carries with it enthusiasm and curiosity embedded on the matrix of creativity. It is through this Energy Release Point that full expression of Free Will, the birthright of our individuality, manifests.

Unblocking and activating this Energy Release Point strengthens vitality and initiative to burst forth and explore life with the natural freedom and curiosity of a child and thereby living a purposeful life. It furthermore assists in releasing childhood trauma, allowing for movement through fear, in order to continue and flow the path of destiny.

Disharmonies: *Fear; anxiety; exhaustion and fatigue; overly serious tendencies; workaholic tendencies; inability to play; lack of spontaneity.*

KID-14 Fullness of Four

Virtues: This Energy Release Point brings together two very important concepts; the number four as well as fullness brought by abundance and plenty. The number four represents movement. In music, intervals of the fourth were used in sacred music of the church inspiring devotion to God and connection through the gift of the Holy Spirit. Humanity has four limbs to move forward, embrace, give and receive the joys that a purposeful life brings. Movement here implies being moved by the joy of Spirit to embrace doing, living and being through our physical vehicle. Four can also be the number for balance, harmony and bringing practicality to our spiritual visions. Nature also provides the number four with producing the winds of the four directions. The winds of change create movement from the four directions and resonantly, nature transforms itself cyclically through the movement of time through the four seasons. In this cyclical movement, humanity is in the centre of the experience. The ability to navigate the movement and changes of life from a state of centre is directly related to one's inner sense of abundance and plenty, as well as being inclusive and generous of nature within grounded practicality. Unblocking and activating this Energy Release Point connects one to centre and balance, allowing the opportunity to penetrate to the inside of our Essence, nourish and fuel vitality, in order to continue forward motion in the fulfillment of desires from a place of abundance.

Disharmonies: *Fear of change; inability to flow with life; fear of lack; miserly or hoarding tendencies; stagnation; inability to serve and give to others. Physical manifestations of bloating; abdominal fullness and distention, gynaecological disorders; fibroids and barrenness.*

KID-16 Vital Centre

Virtues: This Energy Release Point allows one to get to the Heart of the Matter - to explore deeply within one's depths the imbalances of the physical, emotional, mental and spiritual bodies. Often these imbalances present themselves in the form of stomach ailments. Further examination holds that these stomach issues stem back to one's relationship with the feminine. Whether it is a personal relationship with our human mother, or whether it is the acceptance of one's own feminine nature (present in both males and females) or also one's perception of women in society and the value thereof. Simply put, there is a disconnection between our Selves and the Archetypal Divine Mother of the Birthing Feminine Matrix. Unblocking and activating this Energy Release Point allows us to explore these relationships and how we function with them, with this awareness, the flood gates open and a resurgence of new ideas and creativity flow and find their way into our consciousness. This flowing serves to heal our creative centre and through harmonization with the centre of the Divine Feminine Birthing Matrix one gains access to unlimited potential and possibilities of creation.

Disharmonies: *Blocked creativity; lack of vitality; exhaustion in the full body system; digestive disorders leading to depletion; dysfunctional relationship with mother and/or mothering roles; obsessive thinking; anxiety; emotional neediness; insecurity.*

KID-17 Accommodate, Deliberate and Trade / Accommodating Merchant

Virtues: This Energy Release Point metaphorically connects to where we are on our life journey and speaks to the point in the journey where fatigue and weariness can discourage the continuation on the path. It is here where we sit and re-structure, re-align and re-evaluate. This Energy Release Point is the point where we assess our inner qualities and our gifts, as well as the place where we evaluate the ability to assess the quality of our expression. It penetrates inwards to bring forth our unique Essence. Unblocking and activating this Energy Release Point allows us to find the value within, to bend and to be flexible. To be able to make changes within the journey and flow with Spirit. It allows us then to deliberate and trade, to evaluate our resources and know the quality of our worth. Much like the accommodating merchant who replenishes our supplies to continue the journey.

Disharmonies: *Inability to express feelings, especially deep sadness; weariness of life; internalized grief and melancholy. Physical manifestations of intestinal pain and abdominal fullness; no pleasure in eating.*

KID-21 The Dark Hidden Secret Gate

Virtues: This Energy Release Point is the entrance to a dark hidden secret gate. It brings one to an opening into the darkness. It is also to understand that there cannot be a full understanding of darkness without having the experience of seeing light. Also, it is to understand that within even the darkest places, such as the vastness of a night sky with a new moon there are still stars that shine. Within the darkness there is light, within light there is darkness. Walking through the dark gate into the place where emotions and experiences are hidden and forgotten in secrecy allows for the empowerment to transcend fear and to promote flow to joy and freedom. Dark Hidden Secret Gate symbolizes the entry to the burial ground of emperor- the mausoleums, a place of great reverence. Likewise going inwards to face one's darkness, pain and fear is a journey of healing with reverence. Unblocking and activating this Energy Release Point allows for going into the underworld, into the depths of the heart and to bring illumination. It is introspection, and faith in trusting one's inner knowing and wisdom.

Disharmonies: *Inability to face fears; escapism behaviour; searching for external sources for reassurance; over-dependent on others, emotional co-dependence. Physical manifestations of bloating; heaviness; digestive issues.*

Portraits of the Energy Release
Points for the Extraordinary Release
Channel of the Vessel of Guidance

Opening Point

GB-41 Near to Tears

Virtues: This Energy Release Point acknowledges the expressions of frustration and anger so that it can be released. The original pictogram of this Energy Release Point is that of a man on the edge of a cliff, signifying danger. This image, in itself, speaks to the importance of the healthy release of frustration and anger, so that a dangerous situation, either to oneself or to another, does not manifest. Near to Tears brings energy to the expression of healthy tears so that one can move forward, find courage, and make decisions that benefit the health of the Being and relationships with others. It assists in healing areas of darkness and shadows where repressed anger stews, waiting for the opportunity to burst forth. It brings healthy tears that function to relieve stress, especially when one is feeling frustrated and thwarted at every turn. This Energy Release Point is the master point in the Horizontal Vessel of Guidance (Girdle Vessel), which serves as an energetic belt to hold one together. Unblocking and activating this Energy Release Point assists in the release of stress so that one can feel reconnected to purposeful action towards Soul evolution and fulfillment of destiny.

Disharmonies: *Frustration; lack of fulfillment; stress; anger; hysterical behaviour.*

Balance Point

TH-5 Outer Frontier Gate

Virtues: As this is a gate Energy Release Point, it speaks to the importance of harmony between the known inner realms and the unknown outer realms. In order for one to safely navigate the unknown, the feelings of security, safety and connection to inner truth needs to be firmly established within so that it may translate with confidence to the exterior. This gate function also translates to the ease and confidence one feels to embrace living life and participating in the social network. To feel joy in the companionship with others is energizing for the Soul. Unblocking and activating this Energy Release Point allows for discernment of who we extend ourselves to and with whom we do not in accordance with our highest good and wellbeing.

Disharmonies: *To erect barriers towards others; to have dysfunctional boundaries within relationships; social alienation; avoidance of intimacy; embarrassment; feelings of shame; low vitality; premature aging; compromised immunity; extreme fluctuations in temperatures within the body. (For example Reynaud's syndrome, hot flashes.)*

Crossing Points

GB-26 Girdling Vessel of Vital Circulation

Virtues: This Energy Release Point activates forward motion which is steady and balanced, yet joyously enthusiastic. It embraces the sensory experiences of life to the fullest expression. Breathing in experiences, sights and sounds as well as tasting smelling and seeing the world in all it's gloriousness. It is through this Energy Release Point that one connects to the merging of the Soul with the physical vehicle. It creates expansion and regulates the flow of energy between the Cosmos and the Earth within the human body. Unblocking and activating this Energy Release Point is tantamount to lighting up an energy grid that powers up and creates a network of organization that puts life plans into action. Physically, this point is located on the waist, a place where traditionally money belts or coin purses as well as swords were carried. Symbolically, this refers to forward movement on the journey, free from fear, trusting that the necessary resources are in place and available for the adventure of life.

Disharmonies: *Stagnation caused by fear; immobility; paralysis; devitalization; physical manifestation of shingles.*

GB-27 Fifth Pivot

Virtues: This Energy Release Point has the meaning of being one of the five Energy Release Points that function as a pivot point. (ST- 25 Celestial Pivot, GB-28 Maintain the Way, DMD-5 Suspended Pivot, DMD-7 Balanced Central Pivot). Fifth Pivot anchors strength and balance within one's centre through periods of growth, great activity, transformation and change. It is a central pivot around which everything turns. A pivot is an immovable reference point of great calm and stability. It is to be in the centre of great action and activity, transformation and change. Unblocking and activating this Energy Release Point strengthens the ability to rotate flexibly around this central axis. It empowers a strong sense of self, which is balanced within group consciousness, so that one remains flexible and receptive in group work. It promotes decisiveness in thought, and flexibility in action, in order to bring into completion the manifestation of creative energy.

Disharmonies: *Inflexibility and rigidity of mind and body; low sense of self-worth; weak-willed; dysfunctional in group settings; over-attachment to personal will; easily overwhelmed by details; inability to formulate clear goals and plans.*

GB-28 Maintain the Way

Virtues: This Energy Release Point maintains the commitment to walk the path with clear intention and flowing flexibility. To walk the path is to trust in the fundamental unknowability of life and to have confidence to meet the unknown. To have clear commitment to walk the path, one needs clear connection to the will forces of the third energy centre. The third energy centre carries authentic power as derived from the alignment with Divine Will. It embodies the qualities of courage, faith, initiative, dependability, self-reliance and certainty. Walking the path magnetizes and radiates positive consciousness. This Energy Release Point is also a connecting point with the Horizontal Vessel of Guidance (The Belt Vessel). As such, it harmonizes and integrates all decisions and goals made to walk and live a balanced life. It serves to join together all disparate ideas and parts into a synthesized wholeness for purposeful action and mandalic consciousness. This living wholeness allows for the circulation of vital energy which fuels the generation of new ideas, further empowering flexibility within the birthing process to sift and sort through all the possibilities and move into appropriate directions for continual growth and manifestation. Unblocking and activating this Energy Release Point strengthens the commitment to walk the path. It sustains the energy of desire to become the feet, hands and heart of the Divine. Through being a living example of one who understands and lives "The Way", the ability for love and light to flow through the veil and touch the hearts and minds of humanity is magnified.

Disharmonies: *Feelings of constriction and restriction; inability to stay focused and on course; disempowerment; disconnected to purpose and vision; inability to follow through on intention. Physical manifestation of uterine problems; lower abdominal pain; lower back pain; unexplained water swellings; intestinal difficulties.*

LIV-13 Chapter Gate / Completion Gate

Virtues: This Energy Release Point is suggestive of being at the end of a transitory state - where all things complete, where one witnesses and acts upon the turning of a new leaf and moves forward into the next phase of life. Standing in the middle of the gate is not comfortable. From this Point one may choose to go backwards and dwell in the past, perhaps re-writing or re-cycling repetitive thoughts creating worry and stagnation. Or, one may choose to step towards new life experiences. Unblocking and activating this Energy Release Point dissolves walls that block vision and empowers the letting go of old injuries so that one may take the forward step and experience a healthy transition. It also unblocks creativity, allowing for free flow of written work and other artistic pursuits.

Disharmonies: *Frustration; stagnation; nostalgic holding onto the past; resentments; repetitive thought patterns; inability to form visions or goals; inability to keep things in perspective.*

Portraits of the Energy Release Points
for the Extraordinary Release Channel
of the Feminine Vessel of Movement

Opening Point

KID-6 Sea of Reflection and Illumination

Virtues: This Energy Release Point connects to the depths of the vast ocean of consciousness, the womb of creation, where the divine feminine births and generates the potentialities of the Soul. The sea is the microcosm to the ocean and the individual is the microcosm to the sea. The individual, therefore, is made of consciousness - as generated by the Divine Feminine and made active by the Divine Masculine. The oceans, seas, and water systems move and flow by this dynamic energy. The water itself is a reflection of both aspects of the Creative Force - for it holds depth and moisture of primordial being-ness and yet reflects light and activity of the sun, the moon and the stars as active expression of doing-ness. It is inner vitality of inner wisdom. Unblocking and activating this Energy Release Point creates the opportunity to witness the reflection of Soul self brilliance. A brilliance fuelled by illumination and wisdom. By connecting to this brilliance, the mind is illuminated to the unknown nature of Self, in all aspects - the gifts, the beauty, the fears; all that which is buried. It enables conscious connection, allowing reflection into wisdom and thereby healing and releasing that which hinders the full growth into a Self Realized Being.

Disharmonies: *Fear stemming from Karmic sources; shock; trauma; anxiety; feelings of urgency; easily overwhelmed by life circumstances.*

Balance Point

LU-7 Broken Sequence

Virtues: This Energy Release Point empowers the function of receiving inner clarity and letting go; surrendering that which no longer serves. It speaks to the Universal Principle that all is rhythm. We receive and let go. We take in and we move out; everything is rhythmic and everything has an ebb and flow. When we seek to control or stop the rhythm, the sequence or Divine order of things seems broken and chaos ensues. The empowerment of activating this point is a return to balance by strengthening clarity of the concept of detachment and finding centre.

Disharmonies: *Lack of clarity; feelings of loss and longing stemming from childhood; difficulty with letting go and moving forward. Physical disharmonies can manifest as things interrupted or out of rhythm: menstrual cycles, sleep cycles, eating disorders.*

Crossing Points

KID-2 Blazing Valley / Dragon in the Abyss

Virtues: This Energy Release Point evokes the image of fires blazing in a valley. Valleys are usually seen as places of lush green growth and coolness, often within the shadow of the mountains. This Energy Release Point is blazing, it is as though the dragon within the abyss has been poked or jabbed awake from it's slumber and it now rises upwards, breathing it's fire, making his presence known. Unblocking and activating this Energy Release Point unleashes the fire of the dragon. It is highly creative, transformational, magical energy with the ability to harmonize the heart with its flaming passion with our wisdom as embodied by water - the source of the lush valley and the womb of the Divine Feminine. Alchemically, the dragon draws spiritual potency from these seeming opposites. In Ancient texts such as the Wang Fu in China (c.76-163 BC) it is written: Dragon fire and human fire are opposite. If dragon fire comes into contact with wetness it flames; and if it meets water it burns. If one drives it away by means of fire, it stops burning and it's flames are extinguished. Blazing Valley/Dragon in the Abyss is therefore the vision of seeing a dragon emerge from a primal whirlpool in full magnificence and strength. It is the foundation of health and immunity. It empowers illumination into our depths and redirects our consciousness to innate purpose and drive to fulfill destiny.

Disharmonies: *Introversion; depletion; exhaustion from over-striving.*

KID-6 Sea of Reflection and Illumination

Virtues: This Energy Release Point connects to the depths of the vast ocean of consciousness, the womb of creation, where the Divine Feminine births and generates the potentialities of the Soul. The sea is the Microcosm to the ocean and the individual is the Microcosm to the sea. The individual, therefore, is made of consciousness - as generated by the Divine Feminine and made active by the Divine Masculine. The oceans, seas, and water systems move and flow by this dynamic energy. The water itself is a reflection of both aspects of the Creative Force - for it holds depth and moisture of primordial being-ness and yet reflects light and activity of the sun, the moon and the stars as active expression of doing-ness. It is inner vitality of inner wisdom. Unblocking and activating this Energy Release Point creates the opportunity to witness the reflection of Soul self brilliance. A brilliance fuelled by illumination and wisdom. By connecting to this brilliance, the mind is illuminated to the unknown nature of Self, in all aspects - the gifts, the beauty, the fears; all that which is buried. It enables conscious connection, allowing reflection into wisdom and thereby healing and releasing that which hinders the full growth into a Self Realized Being.

Disharmonies: *Fear stemming from Karmic sources; shock; trauma; anxiety; feelings of urgency; easily overwhelmed by life circumstances.*

KID-8 Sincerity and Trust

Virtues: This Energy Release Point creates the pathway of connection to truth, sincerity and trust. It helps build faith and inner wisdom within self and empowers the ability to trust that our communication and exchanges with others will be met with an equal measure of sincerity and truth. This

Energy Release Point creates the environment for harmonious exchange where wisdom prevails and the building of security, commitment, strength, integrity, confidence, sincerity and trust flourishes. Unblocking and activating this Energy Release Point brings peace and harmony to replace the fear which hinders the ability to trust in the communication of our truths and to have confidence that these truths will be well received by those around us. It empowers commitment to manifest our purpose in life as communicated by heaven at the point of our conception, as well as strengthening faith in the outcomes.

Disharmonies: *Fear; anxiety; lack of confidence; expecting the worst in people and in situations; mistrust of others; betrayal issues.*

ST-12 Broken Bowl

Virtues: This Energy Release Point assists in reconstructing that which is shattered. This shattering of the energy field and emotional body can occur when one experiences great loss and remains in illusion and victim consciousness. This state of emotional pain or shatter comes from having poured oneself so completely into another that the integrity of one's wholeness cannot withstand the void of emptiness. This can come from endings of dysfunctional, co-dependent relationships of all kinds. (Parent/child, husband/wife, romantic relationships, and friendships for example). Unblocking and activating this Energy Release Point assists in moving through grief and loss. It assists in raising the consciousness from a personal ego centre to a transcendent larger picture. Moving pain into the heart space to be transformed to joy, to release suffering into re-birth. This transformational point assists in detachment and viewing the larger perspective. To see transition and change as an opportunity for growth; growth filled with enthusiasm of the new life experience which awaits. Empowerment of emotional freedom and unconditional love so that Soul evolution can continue in a self sufficient way.

Disharmonies: *Neediness; co-dependency; worry; drama filled relationships; empty nest syndrome; stage parent; control issues; intense grief;*

victim consciousness; personal attachment; loss of self; loss of individual-
ity; inappropriate boundaries between parents and children. Physically
this point impacts milk production for breast feeding, symbolizing self care,
nurturance; teaching healthy boundaries to the baby and bonding. Improper
bonding creates distrust of the world; instability of one's centre, growing into
a dysfunctional adult. The inability to provide for oneself the nourishment
needed affecting the ability to be self sufficient. (Physically, mentally, emo-
tionally and spiritually). Life is shattered, the illusion is broken and one falls
to pieces.

ST-9 Welcoming Humanity as Part of All

Virtues: This Energy Release Point embodies the principle that "ALL
is in the ALL" and "The ALL is in ALL". It is the unity of consciousness.
The awareness that humanity is a part of nature, that nature is a part of
Heaven, Earth and Humanity. Humanity, therefore, is the totality of the
ALL. Connecting with this Energy Release Point connects us with our
centre where we feel communion and belonging to the Earth. A sense
of home, a sense of support, a unification with all that surrounds us. We
feel connected and in union, and this feeling energizes and boosts vitality.
Unblocking and activating this Energy Release Point provides the opening
to receive and feel the great connection with the Universal ALL. A connection which brings great welcome and joyous connection to Essence. The
connection with Essence clears and empowers vision and enables one to
stand upright with dignity so that the ability to set appropriate boundaries
regarding giving is empowered. It fuels Heart's desire to open, cultivate
compassion, revive generosity of sharing and receiving so that life is filled
with beauty and enriched with abundance. This Energy Release Point furthermore acts to help distinguish one's own needs from those of others,
therefore releasing dysfunctional relationships and re-harmonizing to the
Divine Feminine Mother who nourishes and supports in a healthy way.

Disharmonies: *Isolation; hardened heart; lack of joy; lack of love; lack of*
desire; feeling unsupported; disconnected from spirit; narrow scope of vision;
paranoid; antagonistic projection; misperception of reality; inability to grow,

change or move forward; inability to say no; resentment resulting from habitual giving; ingratiation; hiding our true intentions in order to avoid conflict; co-dependence; neediness.

UB-1 Eyes Full of Illumination

Virtues: This Energy Release Point assists us in discerning the difference between looking and seeing. It opens up the mind's eye and the spiritual eye in order to form clear perceptions of reality, free from judgment and limitation. When one begins to observe what is around them, then one can begin to describe what is seen. This strengthens the ability to be present, really beginning to see and observe for the first time, and then, beginning to see more and more. The wise one will begin to observe and describe the beauty of what is seen. Therefore, the more one sees, connects and holds the description of beauty in the mind's eye - the more the eyes will open with wonder and awe. The eyes begin to fill with illuminated consciousness to see the radiance of the Creative Force in all things. Unblocking and activating this Energy Release Point allows our eyes to open and be filled with the brightness of Spirit. It allows for the alchemy of transforming our vision through the insights and connection to the Spiritual Alchemist's work of creating a golden elixir. It is illumination, compassion and radiance. It brings clarity and wisdom into perfect balance. From this, we are energized and more capable of greeting each day with enthusiasm and vitality.

Disharmonies: *Misperception of reality; distortions of truth; fear; depression.*

Portraits of the Energy Release Points
for the Energy Release Channel of
the Masculine Vessel of Movement

Opening Point

UB-62 Extended Vessel / Ghost Road

Virtues: This Energy Release Point assists in creating the space and containment required to receive, store and circulate higher wisdom and knowledge. It helps with discernment to see what is truth and how this truth is reflected in our life. To discern how we can weed out non-beneficial influences, release extraneous non-serving distractions and to retain the jewel of what is essential to the unfoldment of our life plan. The ability to receive and access Universal Truths and to consciously understand them becomes the blueprint and basis for beneficial co-creative action. Extended Vessel provides a container of resources so that we create a fulfilling life in which we not only develop our wisdom, but also transform our wisdom and Universal Truths through the extension of ourselves into the world by our acts of service to others. Unblocking and activating this Energy Release Point empowers receptivity and allows these wisdoms to flow into us and be held within stores of containment for use towards manifestation of an empowered life. In this way, we are facilitated to become conscious directors of life as well as express ourselves in service to others. As the name Ghost Road suggests, this Energy Release Point is a ghost point. It serves to release negative energies that disconnect one from inner truth, willpower and the directives of the Soul as well as blocking the ability to pay attention to the needs of the body.

Disharmonies: *Fatigue; depression; inflexibility; rigidity in the body; over-striving; inability to access clear focused thoughts. Physical manifestations of pain in the shoulders from over pushing and over work.*

Balance Point

SI-3 Back Ravine

Virtues: This Energy Release Point brings the flexibility needed to over-come obstacles which block one from staying on their course. There are many paths to connection to Soul purpose and vision, and regardless of which path we choose, the goal is to arrive at the final destination. Back Ravine brings flexibility to the process and assists in the navigation of life. It strengthens inter-dependence and clarity, allowing for the discernment to know how, and when, to ask for assistance in order to create situations of positive outcome. It strengthens trust in the Divine plan. Unblocking and activating this Energy Release Point empowers trust. A trust that comes from the connection to our inner wisdom and intuition. A trust that evolves from the practice of discernment and alignment to Truth. As one re-connects with Soul Purpose, the natural outcome is that the physi-cal body benefits by being nourished from within. Back Ravine builds strong forces of vital energy, by generating the continual flow of trust when walking the path.

Disharmonies: *Lack of clarity; untapped forces of masculine forthrightness; lack of vitality.*

Crossing Points

UB-61 Servant's Aid / Quieting of Evil

Virtues: This Energy Release Point is the seventh point from the extremity of the Energy Release Channel of the Urinary Bladder. It is also, numeri-cally, a number seven as it is the sixty first Energy Release Point of the Urinary Bladder. (6 + 1) The number seven is symbolic of pushing us to the next higher level of consciousness/awareness, a number of going boldly forward in the exploration of the unknown. The number seven is composed of two lines. The first line is horizontal. It represents stability and support as well as a view of the unlimited horizon. The potential of all that there is ahead of us in the journey waiting for exploration. The second line is diagonal, representing the freedom of limitation and the courage to follow one's unique path and destiny. The diagonal coming from the stability of the horizontal allows for a clear directed vision of the path. It is a deliberately drawn and manifested creation of direction. Unblocking and activating this Energy Release Point gives the strength to continue onto our destination. It is the strength of a faithful servant, one who nourishes and supports the ability to stay on the path, bringing the strength of unwavering conviction of the inner being of the lifestream so that one can express and live purposefully. Within this strength of the journey, there is an understanding, a commitment to oneself and the Divine which reassures safety, trust and success. It is the unfoldment of a perfect Life-power, where one knows that the logical consequence of the unfoldment of ideas and plans will triumphantly manifest as they are meant to. The idea and the plan in itself is a perfect creation. As the name Quieting of Evil suggests, it releases the influences and limitations imposed by errant thought forms that torment the mind and distract one from connecting to authenticity and the vision of the Soul. It dispels enchantments, illusions and spells that cause great fear.

Disharmonies: *Undertakings that frequently fail in their final steps before completion- due to fear; attracting thought forms which perpetuate fear; easily influenced by others, thereby losing connection with authenticity and inner truth; entity invasion/possession.*

UB-59 To Access Masculine Energy

Virtues: This Energy Release Point speaks to the ability of accessing strong, forthright movement and action. Energy that is strongly associated with masculine power. Unblocking and activating this energy Release Point creates the movement to stir up, expose and release stagnation due to toxicity. This is likened to a strong light which serves to find and expose that which is hidden, bring it to awareness in order for it to be removed. To Access Masculine Energy assists in maintaining flowing active energy which serves to keep clear and remove environmental, emotional, mental and spiritual toxicity.

Disharmonies: *Attachment to co-dependent relationships; environmental sensitivity; enmeshed in a lifestyle of toxicity; congestion and inflammation in the body; stagnation.*

GB-29 Dwelling in the Strength of the Bone

Virtues: This Energy Release Point empowers the feelings of protection by building the strength of the bones so that structure is maintained. It is here that strength gathers so that dynamic energy can be created. Wellsprings of energy are valuable resources for decision making, for once a decision is made, there must be energy in place for intentional action and concrete manifestation. Sometimes these actions are necessary break away actions. Break away action in that one needs to release themselves from self destructive patterns and lifestyles, or move away from limiting influences such as those found in family, friends or intimate relationships. This Energy Release Point not only finds the courage to follow one's own path and destiny, but assists in connecting to one's inner strength found within the bones. Unblocking and activating this Energy Release Point brings energy towards taking decisive action toward following the path of truth. It provides trust in knowing that the strength necessary to take the beginning steps is abundantly available. It brings centre and support to one's Being so that goals can be flexible within the virtue of positive structure. It further assists with the absolute knowing that one is loved, supported and protected by the spiritual world for the unfoldment of the Soul's journey.

Disharmonies: *Procrastination; inaction based on fear; doubt; confusion; inflexibility. Physical manifestation of disorders in the hip; lower back pain; atrophy in the legs.*

SI-10 Shoulder Blade

Virtues: This Energy Release Point is named for it's geographical location of the shoulder blade. It is the meeting point of the Energy Release Channel of the Small Intestine, the Extraordinary Energy Release Channel of the Masculine Vessel of Movement and the Extraordinary Energy Release Channel of the Masculine Vessel of Structure. The resulting benefit of this Energy Release Point therefore speaks to the creation of an energy which is greater than the sum of its parts. It is the ability to shoulder the responsibilities of life and helps one to stand in a strong and erect manner. It is stability and centre and as such, keeps everything in balance, nourishing the health of the physical body. It opens a conduit which flows a dynamic source of vitality. It serves to circulate this vitality through the body so that one successfully accomplishes one's mission, reminding us that the Soul is immortal and we are here to share our gifts in service to the elevation of consciousness of humanity. Unblocking and activating this Energy Release Point increases life energy so that one can encounter situations with confidence. It assists in balancing one's unique individuality with the energy of group consciousness so that one can function in wholeness within a larger social matrix.

Disharmonies: *Blocks the free flow of energy of the Secondary Energy Centre of the shoulder.*

LI-15 Shoulder Majesty

Virtues: This Energy Release Point addresses the ability to shoulder responsibility in a strong and capable manner. The name Shoulder Majesty invokes the image of dignity, strength, self empowerment, healthy self esteem and Mastery. A well run kingdom has the qualities of strong management and clarity, working for the benefit of the people. The shoulder is located between the mind and the heart and serves as intermediary. It integrates the clarity of what needs to be done with the forces of the heart, empowering compassion and love based service. It allows for clear discernment and strengthens the ability to respond to what is to be let go and what is to be retained. Unblocking and activating this Energy Release Point strengthens the ability to shoulder responsibility and release feelings of burden. It helps to extend oneself in heart-based service to humanity. It further empowers one to surrender, ask for, and accept the assistance of others when necessary.

Disharmonies: *Over-striving beyond one's limits leading to physical exhaustion; unyielding; inability to ask and/or receive help from others; martyrdom; continual rescuing behaviour; hero complex.*

LI-16 Great Bone

Virtues: This Energy Release Point has two important aspects within the name - the noun Bone and its adjective Great. Bones, in and of themselves, are the structure of the body. They are the foundation of where we have come from. Within the bones, are the memories of our experiences as well as those of our genetic lineage, flowing within the bone marrow. Our foundation and structure of the bones create the shape of our body. Within the foundation and structure of the bones - our bone marrow, genetic lineage, family, cultural traditions and our values, create the shape of our lives. Within all this is the Seed Memory of the gift of being created. The remembrance of the Great Soul Within. The Soul has great work to do. It is said that great work requires great intensity and Soul passion. This Energy Release Point calls us to our Mastery. Mastery assists in the release of that which blocks the cultivation of our gifts. It empowers the ability to stand tall, with dignity and healthy esteem born of our worthiness. In this way, the strength required to shoulder our responsibilities flow with ease from the foundation of our bones. Unblocking and activating this Energy Release Point reminds one of the greatness within, our worthiness and the realization of the importance of what we bring to the world.

Disharmonies: *Low self worth; feelings of unimportance; contempt; bitterness; overwhelmed by duties and responsibilities; structural aches in the shoulders and neck.*

ST-9 Welcoming Humanity as Part of ALL

Virtues: This Energy Release Point embodies the principle that "ALL is in the ALL" and "The ALL is in ALL". It is the unity of consciousness. The awareness that humanity is a part of nature, that nature is a part of Heaven, Earth and Humanity. Humanity, therefore, is the totality of the ALL. Connecting with this Energy Release Point connects us with our centre where we feel communion and belonging to the Earth. A sense of home, a sense of support, a unification with all that surrounds us. We feel connected and in union, and this feeling energizes and boosts vitality. Unblocking and activating this Energy Release Point provides the opening to receive and feel the great connection with the Universal ALL. A connection which brings great welcome and joyous connection to Essence. The connection with Essence clears and empowers vision and enables one to stand upright with dignity so that the ability to set appropriate boundaries regarding giving is empowered. It fuels Heart's desire to open, cultivate compassion, revive generosity of sharing and receiving so that life is filled with beauty and enriched with abundance. This Energy Release Point furthermore acts to help distinguish one's own needs from those of others, therefore releasing dysfunctional relationships and re-harmonizing to the Divine Feminine Mother who nourishes and supports in a healthy way.

Disharmonies: *Isolation; hardened heart; lack of joy; lack of love; lack of desire; feeling unsupported; disconnected from spirit; narrow scope of vision; paranoid; antagonistic projection; misperception of reality; inability to grow, change or move forward; inability to say no; resentment resulting from habitual giving; ingratiation; hiding our true intentions in order to avoid conflict; co-dependence; neediness.*

ST-4 Earth Granary / Earth Greening

Virtues: This Energy Release Point harmonizes the relationships between appetite, need and nourishment. The name itself brings into our consciousness the image of our Earth and it's potential of being an unlimited source of nourishment. In the alternate name, the picture of Earth

Greening speaks of abundance, health, vitality and fertility. Greening is the movement of transformative regenerated energy which is witnessed in the spring. Greening is the word used by the mystic St. Hildegard of Bingen to describe the breath of the Holy Spirit of God giving life to all things. A granary functions as a storage facility. It stores the reserves of nourishment from the harvest and symbolizes abundance and security. Unblocking and activating this Energy Release Point brings into our consciousness the remembrances of knowledge that all is provided. One has what is needed and now can be empowered to assist others. From this realization of abundance, true generosity and altruism are nourished. This Energy Release Point also speaks to our relationship with our mother as a physical embodiment of the greater "Earth Mother" or "Feminine Nurturing Matrix". Ideally, the balanced mother teaches and models for her infants and children, appropriate boundaries in life. Teaching through this balanced identification of herself, bringing the fulfillment of both her needs and the needs of the children. By extension, the needs of the entire family are met and hence assists with the interactions of the individual within the larger community.

Disharmonies: *Selfishness; habitual giving; hoarding tendencies; feelings of not having enough; neediness; inability to receive; disempowerment. Physical manifestations can present as anorexia; bulimia; binge eating; emotional eating; digestive issues; cravings especially for sweets.*

ST-3 Great Hole

Virtues: This Energy Release Point addresses the ability to release excessive thought and worry in order to obtain inner peace. It is the ability to be emotionally honest with oneself, acknowledge emotional pain and remove the mask of cheerfulness used as a coping mechanism when facing the world. It accesses our inner core and provides the strength and courage to deal with the worries that deplete our vitality and compromise mental stability. The physical location of this Energy Release Point is in the hole of the cheek bone. Bones provide structure and protection for the whole body. Unblocking and activating this Energy Release Point brings connection to the inner core of the bones and the centre of one's Being where roots of security and stability are accessed. Strengthening the connection to the bones and centre of Self, strengthens the feelings of stability, security and protection. This flow of vital strength brings courage to the forefront to address emotional pain and the fortitude to continue despite obstacles in the navigation through life. Ultimately, one feels the freedom to live authentically, in positive vulnerability and Soul expression.

Disharmonies: *Worrisome thoughts; having a busy mind; denial and avoidance of emotional pain. Physical manifestations of pain and numbness of the face and lips; toothaches.*

ST-1 Receive Tears / Flowing Tears

Virtues: This Energy Release Point helps to flow emotional congestion in order to understand and receive insightful nourishment from painful experiences. The Soul experiences emotions through the interaction of the emotional body with the physical body. When painful emotions are experienced, there can be a detachment; a coping mechanism. This detachment serves to anesthetize the feeling life. Detachment over time can lead to a false mask of cheerfulness, denial, or addictive behaviours, which ultimately creates congestion in the physical body. This congestion can present not only as digestive issues but also cause body inflammation, particularly in the elimination system and in the sinus cavity. Unblocking and activating this Energy Release Point is similar to opening a floodgate which relieves and cleanses this emotional congestion. Once the congestion is released, it becomes easier to acknowledge and work with emotional pain, receive nourishment and understand the painful aspects of the past. With the re-establishment of flow and movement, reception of wisdom is facilitated as well as the ability to let go is enhanced. In this way, the Soul continues to learn and grow in wisdom and emotional strength.

Disharmonies: *Inability to cry; feeling heavy or oppressed; inability to let go of the past; needy behaviour; manipulation of others through tears.*

UB-1 Eyes Full of Illumination

Virtues: This Energy Release Point assists us in discerning the difference between looking and seeing. It opens up the mind's eye and the spiritual eye in order to form clear perceptions of reality, free from judgment and limitation. When one begins to observe what is around them, then one can begin to describe what is seen. This strengthens the ability to be present, really beginning to see and observe for the first time, and then, beginning to see more and more. The wise one will begin to observe and describe the beauty of what is seen. Therefore, the more one sees, connects and holds the description of beauty in the mind's eye - the more the eyes will open with wonder and awe. The eyes begin to fill with illuminated consciousness to see the radiance of the Creative Force in all things. Unblocking and activating this Energy Release Point allows our eyes to open and be filled with the brightness of Spirit. It allows for the alchemy of transforming our vision through the insights and connection to the Spiritual Alchemist's work of creating a golden elixir. It is illumination, compassion and radiance. It brings clarity and wisdom into perfect balance. From this, we are energized and more capable of greeting each day with enthusiasm and vitality.

Disharmonies: *Misperception of reality; distortions of truth; fear; depression.*

GB-20 Wind Pond

Virtues: This Energy Release Point helps in the navigation of life during times of chaos and upheaval. Wind brings change and during the process of change there is at times destruction and breakdown. Wind Pond has the ability to connect to the vibrant energy of wind and use that energy for the positive implementation of necessary action within the process of transformation and rebirth. It restores orientation, perspective and vibrant mental clarity. It helps one to make decisions and implement plans when faced with unpredictable life circumstances. This Energy Release Point unblocks the thinking life so that consciousness can be activated for higher activity. Higher thinking has the ability to penetrate deep into consciousness in order to reconnect to the essence of dreams and vision of the Soul. In this place of clarity, goals for the fulfillment of life purpose can be strategized and implemented into action. Unblocking and activating this Energy Release Point brings wakeful clarity. Clarity in the way of being keen and alert as though there are eyes on the back of the head. It is mindful and awake consciousness that can draw on the reservoir of wind energy to put life into action.

Disharmonies: *Inability to reconcile what we see in the world with our sense of self; remorse and regrets from the past; constantly changing plans and decisions; inability to deal with life's changing circumstances; sudden anger when needing to alter plans; inability to adapt to present circumstances due to inflexibility; indecisiveness and poor planning. Physically this can manifest as headaches; dizziness; sinus congestion; plugged ears and runny eyes.*

Portraits of the Energy Release Points for the Energy Release Channel of the Feminine Vessel of Structure

Opening Point

P-6 Inner Frontier Gate / Inner Palace Gate

Virtues: This Energy Release Point embodies our journey into our hearts - the frontier and unexplored territory known as the borderlands. The journey into this transition zone cannot help but create transformation - for in the act of undertaking the journey itself one is transformed through the encounter of the unknown. As a gate point, one is empowered to come and go at will understanding the appropriate boundaries in relation to the sanctity of the Heart and sharing oneself with others. Qualities of compassion, connection, warmth and Light are accessed and bring the perseverance to proceed onward with the journey. Unlocking the gate to this inner heart space signifies a profound turning point for the one willing to pass through and transform pain and hurt into blessings of peace and calmness. Unblocking and activating this Energy Release Point can assist in calming the Self from the trauma of betrayal from intimacy, rape, incest or divorce.

Disharmonies: *Closing the heart in self protection from the pain of intimacy; projecting old pain onto the present; feelings of being stabbed or shot in the heart due to betrayal or painful separations.*

Balance Point

SP- 4 Yellow Emperor / Grandparent-Grandchild

Virtues: This Energy Release Point is the only Energy Release Point on the body with a royal name. It speaks to human history that is found in mythology. In this mythology one finds a distant Divine ancestor representing Heaven, as well as a distant ancestor representing Earth. In this respect it serves to unify the light of the mind of Heaven with the passion of the Heart of Earth. It is to be unselfish, to be open to all and to create and share posterity for the benefit of humanity. This Energy Release Point also is the family name of the mythological Yellow Emperor who ruled China for 100 years from 2697 BC to 2597 BC. It is symbolic of gold, royalty, merit, youth, virginity, happiness and fertility. It is the Yellow Emperor that received ancient wisdom of medicine to help ease the suffering of his people. He taught them to be stewards of the Earth and the Earth in turn would nourish the nation. By tending the Earth and teaching future generations the ability to do the same, the Emperor could be assured that prosperity, stability and abundance would be the birthright of all the descendants of his people. In this way, future generations would continually reap the riches of the harvests and as such this would be the inheritance of the royal treasury. Unblocking and activating this Energy Release Point empowers the unification of generations. It forms a bridge between the wisdom of the past and brings hope for the future. It unites and strengthens the ability to act in accordance to the heart's passion while strengthening the forces of will. Yellow Emperor combines strength with wisdom and creates hope and optimism for the future generations in order for humanity to continue the journey.

Disharmonies: *Dysfunctional comfort seeking behaviour; addictions or addictive behaviour; being disheartened and depressed; hopelessness; pessimism and despair; conflict with images of authority; alienation from the past; disconnection with genetic lineage; unconscious wasteful behaviour in regards to environmental issues; disconnection from nature; unconscious exploitative behaviours in regards to nature.*

Crossing Points

KID-9 Building Guest

Virtues: This Energy Release Point strengthens the creativity centre, creating the room for welcoming and housing a baby or for the gestation of a project, or artistic creation. This Energy Release Point empowers the continual flow of life as it takes a seed, gestates it, transforming it for birth. It is a spiritual embryo as well, incubating and awakening us to life and the pursuit of the development of our talents and cultivation of our potential, the birthing of our new self. Unblocking and activating this Energy Release Point begins the process of creating and re-birthing. One cannot conceive solely on one's own. There must be a joining of masculine and feminine energies. Likewise inspiration is received from the exterior and drawn in. The Divine Energy or breath of Spirit brings forward the awakening of creativity and flowering of potential.

Disharmonies: *Infertility on one or more levels of Being: the physical, emotional, mental and spiritual planes. Feeling unsupported; unloved; feeling of lack.*

SP-6 Union of the Three Feminine Mysteries

Virtues: This Energy Release Point enhances three Divine Mysteries: the storage and distribution of Spirit; the connection with Spirit; the Flowing with Spirit. When these three mysteries are brought together for unification and integration, they amplify strength and vibrancy. The number three is symbolic for understanding the components necessary for brilliant creativity. It conveys the idea that through growth found in creative expression, comes perfect manifestation as inspired by the movement of Spirit. Unblocking and activating this Energy Release Point enhances the action of the Three Treasures, that of receiving inspiration of Heaven and mingling it with vitality drawn of the Earth so that passionate energy, fuelled by the Heart of Desire, can evolve and move into full expression of the manifestation of potential.

Disharmonies: *Deep depression; desperation; wanting to run away from a situation, circumstance, people, place or thing; frustration to the point of rebelliousness.*

SP-13 Official Residence, Our Home

Virtues: This Energy Release Point allows for transformation. A healthy and easy transformation which comes from being connected to a stabilized strength of home in the centre of our Being. It promotes harmony and calm allowing for the energy of being present. When one is fully present, one can solidify a vision of creativity and manifest a purpose filled life. Unblocking and activating this Energy Release Point allows one to connect to this place of wellbeing, empowering refinement of the quality of care and nurturance one gives to oneself, as well as strengthening the physical condition of the body.

Disharmonies: *Scattered thinking and an overactive mind; feeling lost like a child and looking for help. Physically this Energy Release Point helps with abdominal fullness and distention, abdominal pain and constipation.*

SP-15 Great Horizontal

Virtues: This Energy Release Point promotes the firmness of support derived from standing on a strong foundation. This foundation is built on life experiences. When one goes through life feeling the support of the masculine in particular, there is an energy of strength and unwavering trust that all will proceed with positive intention for benevolence and joy. Likewise, when this is integrated with the support of the feminine Earth, we are empowered to stand firmly knowing that we are provided for and protected. This ensures healthy self sufficiency. When one integrates both these feminine and masculine aspects, one is rewarded with a renewed sense of vitality. The ability to form healthy boundaries when in service to others and receive the exchange flows naturally and with ease. It can also be said that life experiences can be obscured by the energy of pain. Pain, such as sadness, grief or dysfunctional relationships. Great Horizontal allows us to draw on the strength of a positive foundation in order to eliminate this energy of pain. Connecting to this Energy Release Point brings to awareness the knowledge that the support was always there, for its basis is a Divine Source. It is recognizing that the pain obscured the view. This obscurity is often caused by a dysfunctional relationship to the father or masculine. Through Great Horizontal, one connects to a place where a higher and broader perspective is shown. A place where one can view the horizon at all angles and move in any direction free from past encumbrances brought on by pain and grief. Unblocking and activating this Energy Release Point strengthens the ability to let go of grief in order to make room for vitality. It strengthens the feelings of being supported and loved as well as allows for the development of trust in the masculine.

Disharmonies: *Exhaustion and fatigue; sadness; weeping; sighing; resigned sacrifice of one's own needs for the fulfillment of others; too tired to go on.*

SP-16 Abdomen Sorrow and Lament

Virtues: This Energy Release Point connects into the depths where one finds peace and calm. This is extremely beneficial when life presents experiences of great sorrow such as the loss of a loved one or the loss of a relationship. It allows one to lament and have a passionate expression of grief. It brings compassion and tenderness in times of devastating pain in order to move through distress by flowing tears. Tears must express in order to heal sorrow. Tears serve as a harmonizer and heart balancer. They allow the passage of sorrow so that other emotions can flow in and be experienced. Abdomen Sorrow and Lament is also beneficial for resolution when one feels that they have missed or lost an opportunity. It assists in helping one to release regret and longing for another chance to express what needed to be said in order to find resolution within. Unblocking and activating this Energy Release Point assists in healing the sorrow and distresses in life. It allows for the full expression of distress and emotional pain. It brings a renewal of compassion for Self, strengthens the belief that life continues and that one can trust that needs will once again be met. Through inner peace and calm, connection with spiritual beings and the Divine Source is more easily accessed strengthening the awareness that healing love flows eternal.

Disharmonies: *Deep emotional pain and devastation; grief; longing; loneliness; sorrow; deep seated abandonment and depression; emotional emptiness; inability to see visions of the future thereby blocking creativity and forward motion. Physical manifestations of emotional pain showing as noisy intestines; anxiety; infertility; eating disorders; wasting diseases; weeping body showing as diarrhea.*

LIV-14 Gate of Hope / Expectation's Door

Virtues: This Energy Release Point empowers hope and the quality of aspiration. We aspire to fulfill our purpose, and are inspired and drawn onward toward the highest potential in our life. Perceived obstacles are dissolved and we are empowered to find creative solutions with renewed optimism. To take action based on our commitments and goals. Being in the NOW. Living in the moment is considered to be very healthy, yet it does pose a fine balance - that of the inability to see into the future, yet to trust that all is going to proceed in a healthy, happy way. Within this element of trust there is balance, for it is the recognition and living co-creatively with the Creative Force. Through this co-creativity, clarity of vision is enhanced. When vision is clear, purpose becomes clearer. From this perspective one can allow for planning and foresight, as well as goal setting and achievement. All by being fully present in the NOW. The best decisions and plans therefore, are those which are harmonious and in alignment with one's purpose and Higher Self, thereby creating the feeling and appearance of free-flow, the virtues of ease and grace within manifestation of dreams and vision.

Disharmonies: *Hopelessness; mental torture; suicidal tendencies; apathy; internalized anger; melancholia; negativity and irritability; unrealistic expectations leading to disappointment; procrastination derived from the belief of having time in the future which prevents initiation of meaningful change.*

DFM-22 Celestial Chimney, the Opening of the Heavens

Virtues: This Energy Release Point is located in the notch of the sternum at the base of the neck. It is a beautiful window or passageway that allows for the flowing movement of Spirit. It allows a connection between our body, which may feel heavy and oppressed, to the Universal Mind of the Creative Force. The passageway between Heaven and Earth. This Energy Release Point reminds us to evaluate our relationship to the masculine: our Solar aspects, our fathers, brothers and partners. It helps us to break through patterns of diminishment, severe mood changes, impetuous, unexpected self-destructive behaviours or situations. Celestial Chimney, The Opening of the Heavens is a conduit to the return to clarity from experiences of shock, fear or trauma. Unblocking and activating this Energy Release Point allows for a clear passage and facilitates the ability to express from the core of our Being. It strengthens the ability of clear thinking, reception of inspiration and enthusiasm. It reminds one to breathe and flow with the Universal breath. It empowers the dispersal of stagnation and forward movement through the realization that you may surrender to where you are in this present moment, even when in pain. Through the act of surrendering, pain is transmuted into forgiveness and release.

Disharmonies: *Asthma; bronchitis; sore and swollen throat; excess mucus and laboured breathing; inability to swallow food; oversensitivity to the remarks and observations of others; throwing up life; inability to accept life and life situations; stiffness of the tongue; inability to express; swelling of the back of the neck.*

DFM-23 Majesty's Spring

Virtues: This Energy Release Point speaks to the purity and vitality of a source of fresh spring water, bubbling up in confidence, freshness and clarity. This water springs forth from the Earth and carries within it's consciousness, the memories of knowledge, skills and talents derived from the experience of the journey. It empowers the view of perspective and the ability to look at life from all angles. This spring bursts through the Earth as a true embodiment of joy, humbled yet honoured to carry the consciousness of knowledge and wisdom. Unblocking and activating this Energy Release Point connects us to the Majesty's Spring source of purity, where we humbly recognize the brilliant sparkle of who we are and allow Light to shine into our crystal depths. It supports us to live our life and step into our majestic mastery so our ability to expand and share our knowledge, skills and talents with others is renewed with a freshness that gives our life meaning.

Disharmonies: *Constant seeker; thirsting for more due to our perceived inadequacies; lack of ideas; verbal dryness; loss of voice due to not wanting to be heard; lack of confidence; holding back our potential.*

Portraits of the Energy Release Points
for the Energy Release Channel of
the Masculine Vessel of Structure

Opening Point

TH-5 Outer Frontier Gate

Virtues: As this is a gate Energy Release Point, it speaks to the importance of harmony between the known inner realms and the unknown outer realms. In order for one to safely navigate the unknown, the feelings of security, safety and connection to inner truth needs to be firmly established within so that it may translate with confidence to the exterior. This gate function also translates to the ease and confidence one feels to embrace living life and participating in the social network. To feel joy in the companionship with others is energizing for the Soul. Unblocking and activating this Energy Release Point allows for discernment of who we extend ourselves to and with whom we do not in accordance with our highest good and wellbeing.

Disharmonies: *To erect barriers towards others; to have dysfunctional boundaries within relationships; social alienation; avoidance of intimacy; embarrassment; feelings of shame; low vitality; premature aging; compromised immunity; extreme fluctuations in temperatures within the body. (For example Reynaud's syndrome, hot flashes)*

Balance Point

GB-41 Near to Tears

Virtues: This Energy Release Point acknowledges the expressions of frustration and anger so that it can be released. The original pictogram of this Energy Release Point is that of a man on the edge of a cliff, signifying danger. This image, in itself, speaks to the importance of the healthy release of frustration and anger, so that a dangerous situation, either to oneself or to another, does not manifest. Near to Tears brings energy to the expression of healthy tears so that one can move forward, find courage, and make decisions that benefit the health of the Being and relationships with others. It assists in healing areas of darkness and shadows where repressed anger stews, waiting for the opportunity to burst forth. It brings healthy tears that function to relieve stress, especially when one is feeling frustrated and thwarted at every turn. This Energy Release Point is the master point in the Horizontal Vessel of Guidance (Girdle Vessel), which serves as an energetic belt to hold one together. Unblocking and activating this Energy Release Point assists in the release of stress so that one can feel reconnected to purposeful action towards Soul evolution and fulfillment of destiny.

Disharmonies: *Frustration; lack of fulfillment; stress; anger; hysterical behaviour.*

Crossing Points

UB-63 Golden Gate / Bridge Pass

Virtues: This Energy Release Point brings one to the place of ultimate safety. When one feels safe, there is security, calmness and peace. These conditions are necessary in order to receive the subtle messages of the Soul, messages which will assist in promoting a balanced flow in all aspects of life. A bridge is a structure which provides a connection between two different things. On the physical level, there are examples of bridges connecting two opposites sides of a river. In this function of connection, the bridge provides safe passage. There are, however, many aspects to a bridge. On the emotional/mental level, a bridge provides support through times of distress so that the state of calm can be restored. On the spiritual level, the bridge provides the state of ease and grace, protection and guidance during threshold experiences. It is connection with the golden light of Christ Consciousness. Golden Gate is a reference to mythology, where there is a mysterious queen mother of the West in the land of the setting sun. She is pictured as a golden gate that welcomes the souls of those who are entering the stage of completion of their life journey on the physical plane. She is beautiful, calm and loving. She baths them with her golden life giving waters so that the souls are refreshed and renewed for the next stage of their journey - re-birth into the spirit world. Unblocking and activating this Energy Release Point opens the sensory orifices for better reception of Divine messages. It promotes the ability to feel the guidance and protection of the spiritual world so that one feels ultimate safety and trust in the unfoldment of life. Perception and awareness is enhanced. Access to the flow of life giving waters brings regeneration and rejuvenation of energy, so that the ability to align with the universal rhythm of life expresses with ease and grace.

Disharmonies: *Stagnation caused by fear of the unknown; inability to embrace life due to fear; anxiety; agitated mind; overwhelm; feeling of drowning in responsibilities and life circumstances; spiritual orphan; feeling cut off from guidance; fear of death.*

GB-35 Masculine Intersection

Virtues: This Energy Release Point creates a network of harmony that unites the flow of masculine energy within the body. This fullness of flow can then direct power for the circulation of light force energy throughout the full body systems for well balanced growth. This Energy Release Point connects to the Masculine Vessel of Structure (Yang Wei Mai) whose function is to stabilize structure and to harmonize the body during times of change and periods of growth. In this way, it communicates the virtues of equilibrium and balance within the Universal Laws. Unblocking and activating this Energy Release Point promotes communication of energy with the masculine aspects of self. It balances distortions or vacillations of self within the context of the ability to harness and unify powerful masculine energy for action and completion of goals.

Disharmonies: *Distorted sense of self which erodes Soul expression; belief systems which undermine the ability to feel success or achievement;*

communication issues; strong ego with narcissism. Physical manifestation of knee inflammation; sciatic pain; pain and cold in the lower leg and foot; asthma and pain in the chest.

GB-29 Dwelling in the Strength of the Bone

Virtues: This Energy Release Point empowers the feelings of protection by building the strength of the bones so that structure is maintained. It is here that strength gathers so that dynamic energy can be created. Wellsprings of energy are valuable resources for decision making, for once a decision is made, there must be energy in place for intentional action and concrete manifestation. Sometimes these actions are necessary break away actions. Break away action in that one needs to release themselves from self destructive patterns and lifestyles, or move away from limiting influences such as those found in family, friends or intimate relationships. This Energy Release Point not only finds the courage to follow one's own path and destiny, but assists in connecting to one's inner strength found within the bones. Unblocking and activating this Energy Release Point brings energy towards taking decisive action toward following the path of truth. It provides trust in knowing that the strength necessary to take the beginning steps is abundantly available. It brings centre and support to one's Being so that goals can be flexible within the virtue of positive structure. It further assists with the absolute knowing that one is loved, supported and protected by the spiritual world for the unfoldment of the Soul's journey.

Disharmonies: *Procrastination; inaction based on fear; doubt; confusion; inflexibility. Physical manifestation of disorders in the hip; lower back pain; atrophy in the legs.*

LI-14 Upper Arm

Virtues: This Energy Release Point connects us to the identity of our True Self and our inner authority as decreed by the Creative Force. In many organizations, the badge of authority is sewn on the upper arm of a jacket. This would be the illusion of outer authority, such as that of high ranking government or military officials, or identities of a cultural group such as the Jewish peoples in World War II. The True Self does not require outer identity or outward signs acknowledging its authority. The True Self has the knowledge and wisdom of the Creative Force through the Connection to the I AM Presence within. This connection ensures the guidance needed to direct one's life in purity, wisdom and heavenly justice. Unblocking and activating this Energy Release Point draws forth the vitality necessary to live a life of courage and authenticity. It empowers living our truth and moving forward in confidence, respect and dignity for self and for others.

Disharmonies: *Grief; longing; control issues especially around relationship; excessive pride; feelings of superiority; prejudice.*

TH-13 Shoulder / Upper Arm Convergence

Virtues: This Energy Release Point renews the abilities of flexibility and reciprocity. It is the ability to perceive and be aware of many points of view in order to assess the next active step. It also allows for harmonious group consciousness, for the ability to listen and take in differing opinions and evaluate options and possible choices. With a flexible mind, the ability to respond to life's demands becomes more balanced. From a balanced perspective, leadership qualities develop and appropriate delegation of tasks to others are facilitated by inspiration and example. Unblocking and activating this Energy Release Point enhances the ability to respond, balances receptivity and cooperation by empowering the ability to give and receive the necessary support in service to others.

Disharmonies: *Inability to ask for assistance; difficulty in sharing tasks leading to overwhelm and inaction; blocked leadership potential; overly intense in leadership. Physically this can manifest in shoulder pain.*

TH-15 Heavenly Crevice / Heavenly Healing

Virtues: This Energy Release Point empowers warmth in the shoulder to assist in extending our heart into the world. When this point is unblocked and activated, it allows for the visualization of what we would see as heaven as well as support this vision and our abilities in bringing this vision into physical manifestation. It is however, more a state of vibrational frequency than a place. When this state is achieved, one can listen, perceive and understand the promptings of the Heart. These Heart promptings speak particularly to our relationship to the masculine energy within, as well as our fathers, brothers and/or intimate partners. Unblocking and Activating this Energy Release Point provides a space of harmony, allowing for a strong flow of Spirit and great transformation.

Disharmonies: *Fear of intimacy and friendships; withdrawal from social engagement; physical manifestations of frozen shoulder; arthritis; pain and stiffness in the neck and arm.*

GB-21 Shoulder Well

Virtues: This Energy Release Point allows for the flow of communication from the Creative Force into our energy field and energy body in order to reach into our physical consciousness. It is through this communication that one can transform the pain of servitude and burden into joyous service. To be able to shoulder responsibilities in a successful and satisfactory way. A way which inspires benevolence, non-judgment and emotional flexibility. It is freedom from servitude. It teaches through example, the necessity of appropriate responses by honouring and respecting the needs of the self. Unblocking and activating this Energy Release Point provides insight into one's assessment of one's ability to respond. It allows for a higher perspective of joy to permeate the tasks that one needs to accomplish. Service to self and others become the expression of vibrant energy flowing from the regenerative properties of the Creative Force.

Disharmonies: *Judgmental attitudes; belligerence; inappropriate anger; constraint. Physically this can manifest as symptoms of tight shoulders and the inability to turn the head - leading to a limited perspective of life.*

SI-10 Shoulder Blade

Virtues: This Energy Release Point is named for it's geographical location of the shoulder blade. It is the meeting point of the Energy Release Channel of the Small Intestine, the Extraordinary Energy Release Channel of the Masculine Vessel of Movement and the Extraordinary Energy Release Channel of the Masculine Vessel of Structure. The resulting benefit of this Energy Release Point therefore speaks to the creation of an energy which is greater than the sum of its parts. It is the ability to shoulder the responsibilities of life and helps one to stand in a strong and erect manner. It is stability and centre and as such, keeps everything in balance, nourishing the health of the physical body. It opens a conduit which flows a dynamic source of vitality. It serves to circulate this vitality through the body so that one successfully accomplishes one's mission, reminding us that the Soul is immortal and we are here to share our gifts in service to the elevation of consciousness of humanity. Unblocking and activating this Energy Release Point increases life energy so that one can encounter situations with confidence. It assists in balancing one's unique individuality with the energy of group consciousness so that one can function in wholeness within a larger social matrix.

Disharmonies: *Blocks the free flow of energy of the Secondary Energy Centre of the shoulder.*

GB-20 Wind Pond

Virtues: This Energy Release Point helps in the navigation of life during times of chaos and upheaval. Wind brings change and during the process of change there is at times destruction and breakdown. Wind Pond has the ability to connect to the vibrant energy of wind and use that energy for the positive implementation of necessary action within the process of transformation and rebirth. It restores orientation, perspective and vibrant mental clarity. It helps one to make decisions and implement plans when faced with unpredictable life circumstances. This Energy Release Point unblocks the thinking life so that consciousness can be activated for higher activity. Higher thinking has the ability to penetrate deep into consciousness in order to reconnect to the essence of dreams and vision of the Soul. In this place of clarity, goals for the fulfillment of life purpose can be strategized and implemented into action. Unblocking and activating this Energy Release Point brings wakeful clarity. Clarity in the way of being keen and alert as though there are eyes on the back of the head. It is mindful and awake consciousness that can draw on the reservoir of wind energy to put life into action.

Disharmonies: *Inability to reconcile what we see in the world with our sense of self; remorse and regrets from the past; constantly changing plans and decisions; inability to deal with life's changing circumstances; sudden anger when needing to alter plans; inability to adapt to present circumstances due to inflexibility; indecisiveness and poor planning. Physically this can manifest as headaches; dizziness; sinus congestion; plugged ears and runny eyes.*

GB-19 Vastness of the Brain

Virtues: This Energy Release Point allows for the thinking mind to open and expand so that it may move into emptiness. In the state of emptiness, the ability of the thinking function to receive inspiration from the Infinite Mind is enhanced. In this way, thoughts flow from the Infinite Mind to the mind, and manifestation of these thoughts can be guided from the Heart centre. Allowing the thinking mind this vast freedom of thought allows the pathway of Illumination to open, bringing vastness and expansion to the thought process. This empowers clarity of ideas, actions and emotions. Unblocking and activating this Energy Release Point has a direct result on the neurological physical functioning of the brain. It calms the nervous system so that higher thought and illumination is supported at the highest level, empowering an accurate perception of reality.

Disharmonies: *Mental disturbances; delusion; misperception of reality; impracticality; emotional constraint; anger; belligerence; inability to hear or understand messages from higher dimensional beings; headaches; tremors; tinnitus; inability to meditate.*

GB-18 Receiving Spirit

Virtues: This Energy Release Point amplifies the action of moving Spirit from the body, to the heart, and to the mind, in order to connect with Higher Mind and then flow back down into the body. This action, once established, serves to magnetize Spiritual energy and connection to Ascended Beings of Light. It is amplification of prayer, ceremony, reverence and devotion. Unblocking and activating this Energy Release Point allows for the activation of the Spiritual interface, an interface which energizes our full body system to conscious awareness of our nature, our Essence and our purpose. It firmly supports the growth of our potential in co-creation with universal energy and cosmic forces. It strengthens sensitivity, empathetic receptivity and compassion, flowing these qualities to the external and blessing all those who are touched by its healing energy.

Disharmonies: *Spiritual pride; aloofness; insensitivity; lack of perception for consequences of actions; disconnect; illusion of spiritual superiority fed by false light; the perpetual seeker/spiritual junkie.*

GB-17 Upright Living

Virtues: This Energy Release Point lends its energy to support straightforward action and an unbending attitude in alignment with truth and purpose. It empowers desire for illumination and self realization, and assists in structuring goals towards manifestation of living the Soul's vision. It promotes living in a way aligned with the true Essence of one's Divine Self. Unblocking and activating this Energy Release Point nourishes the vision of the True Self. It strengthens the ability to stay in truth, despite exterior influences, by increasing discernment. It develops the virtues of authenticity, integrity and benevolence, so that thought and intention are in alignment with exterior action.

Disharmonies: *Confusion and indecision about life direction; lack of commitment; inauthenticity; feelings of anger and frustration; easily persuaded.*

GB-16 Windows of the Eyes / Arriving to Greatest Glory

Virtues: This Energy Release Point empowers one to aspire to the highest manifestation of potential as directed by the vision of one's Soul Blueprint. It is about moving forward on our journey through life's experiences, learning lessons along the way in continual forward motion. It is to see the path directly in front in a clear, unobstructed view, free from distractions seeking to divert from fulfillment of purpose. This clarity of vision is further empowered by developing compassion for oneself and others so that the virtue of compassion is amplified and exemplified by one's thoughts, speech and action. Unblocking and activating this Energy Release Point raises consciousness, sharpens discernment, empowers forgiveness of self and others so that wisdom from events and experiences, past and present, create a higher perspective and continually serve the growth and evolution of the Soul.

Disharmonies: *Victim consciousness; belief that life is hard, unfair or a struggle; needing to be right; attachments to future expectations; past regrets; inflexibility; self defined by who/what is our exterior: i.e: job, education, family and spouse; attachment to the old story; judgment of self; judgment of others; blame issues.*

GB-15 Head Directed by the Kindness of Tears

Virtues: This Energy Release Point allows one to rise above self judgment, judgment and condemnation from others and empowers the release of tears which come from acknowledging the pain and frustration of the Soul's experience of being blocked from fulfilling its purpose of incarnation. Unblocking and activating this Energy Release Point allows for the positive action towards goals and desires. It empowers kindness and compassion towards self which extends to benevolence towards others. It allows for the flow of compassionate healing tears which serve to soften the heart, allowing for the healing energy of the heart to release and transform pain. This is similar to spring snows and rains that bring the vibrance of growth and greening. Through the release of tears, one can more easily release the old thoughts and fears, the toxic memories and emotions blocked and fuelled by frustration, in order to move forward in clarity of perception as well as in joy. To take action that is in alignment with our True Self, free from judgment.

Disharmonies: *Frustration; self judgment; overly critical with oneself; misperception of reality; victim consciousness; to be on the point of crying however not able to flow the tears.*

GB-14 Pure and Clear Masculine Energy

Virtues: This Energy Release Point accesses the portal of pure masculine energy allowing for a great outflow of vitality. This vitality creates the momentum needed for manifestation of physical action. The strength and power of vitality can be likened to the energy of the sun: life giving, pure, clear and powerful. Unblocking and activating this Energy Release Point brings the energy of a new day, the sunrise, a day of endless possibilities, which flow effortlessly from one action to the next. Pure, clear masculine energy empowers clarity of vision and humility in the full body systems, releasing dysfunctional emotions that blind us from seeing our Essential Self and living our vision.

Disharmonies: *Inability to take straight forward positive action; indecision and lack of clarity; antagonistic projection; jealousy; envy; anger; judgment and arrogance.*

GB-13 Root Spirit

Virtues: This Energy Release Point anchors Soul vision into the physical body so that it can flower into manifestation. When one is living one's vision, the full body system (physical, emotional, mental and spiritual) functions as a harmonious whole. This Energy Release Point stresses the importance of the emotional and mental body in the process of integration between the spiritual and physical bodies. All four bodies work together. It empowers the ability to see and plan the necessary steps to fulfillment of vision, by defining and setting clear goals for achievement of purpose. It empowers a purposeful, joy filled tenacity to continue forward. It is a metaphor of the tree. The tree's roots tap into the water of the earth and through alchemy, integrates the water with the sunlight captured within it's branches. This process transforms the basic elements of water, light and wood into a living form called a tree. Similar to the tree, the energy field of the human draws in living light energy of the solar forces and cycles it through the body to anchor it into the physicality through the energy centres. It is the visual imagery of a being, standing firmly rooted in the earth, with the arms outstretched to the heavens, firmly integrating into physicality supportive energies which nourish the qualities necessary for the manifestation of purpose. Unblocking and activating this Energy Release Point transforms Soul vision into physical manifestation by strengthening the ability to be fully present and grounded in the physical body. It helps in the planning of goals by supporting conscious intention and coherent thinking. It shines clarity in the understanding of the manifestation process by showing the steps necessary to create the strong foundation - the roots - upon which the entire creation is to be supported.

Disharmonies: *Unfocused; disorganized communication; overwhelmed and frustrated by too many ideas.*

Testimonials

I was introduced to the world of energetic release points over 11 years ago through the study of acupressure and Jin Shin Do while attaining my CHHP Diploma. However, it was not until I met Michèle Marie Gervais and became both her client and her student that I realized what tremendous healing Energetic Release Points could bring!

My healing sessions with Michèle along with her many teachings, brought my healing journey to a whole new level! Her incredible knowledge mastery, amazing inner knowing and intuitiveness, as well as her love, wisdom and compassion, gave me the opportunity to heal and grow exponentially on all levels: physically, mentally, emotionally, and spiritually. That is when the true meaning and value of receiving and giving through the integration of "Energetic Release Points" in healing modalities was finally brought home and what an awesome blessing it was and continues to be.

Not only am I able to experience the amazing healing personally, but as a Certified Holistic Health Practioner and Vibrational Sound Healing Practioner, I was given the most valuable healing tool I could ever hope for. By integrating this modality in my healing practice, I have been presented the honour, privilege and blessing to witness the remarkable, peace, joy, hope and wellbeing that it brings to my clients.

I feel incredibly blessed and am forever grateful to Michèle Marie Gervais for bringing me down such an awesome healing path while on my life's journey!

Laura S. Noël - Certified Holistic Health Practitioner, Soundtouch Therapist, Vibrational Sound Healer - Fahler, Alberta

---

"When Michele Marie supports me to bring in Energy Release Points, colourful waves of energy pulse through every aspect of my being, unlocking and releasing what no longer serves. Powerful words of affirmation assist me in bringing in what is relevant to my experiences in this reality."

Jean Strong - Reiki Master - Canmore AB

"The Energy Release Point work, that I have done with Michele has assisted in "opening me up", opening me up to my wholeness as a human be-ing. I celebrate this opportunity to feel whole and complete and to bring myself more fully to each moment. This work has allowed me to develop a deeper understanding of myself and my place in this life and in the world. I feel a renewed inner strength and resilience as I am moved to an increase in my positive self talk as well as my sense of Self. After working with Michele I am feeling increased joy, clarity with regard to my sense of purpose and I am powerfully sensing and trusting my intuition, which has had a deeply positive impact on my life. I am grateful to Michele Gervais for the writing of this book and for sharing her insightful gifts, talents and skills with the world."

Betty Aitken - Medicine Hat AB

"Spiritual Portraits of the Energy Release Points is a great gift of love that Michele Marie freely shares with the World and beyond. Each page holds the opportunity, an invitation you might say to go deeper, to explore and ignite the truth that lies within the DNA of each cell of our being. I am continually amazed at the clarity and wisdom Spiritual Portraits brings to each issue and situation asking to be cleared. I truly feel Michele Marie has created a reference book that will stand the test of time always remaining current in the years and centuries to come."

Georgina Grayston -TFT Practitioner - Edmonton AB

"Nearly a decade ago I began seeking help for a scent-sensitivity. On a hunch, I walked into Michele's office and I've known her as my teacher ever since. Her guidance and wisdom first with Soundtouch and the Colourtouch work is what helped awaken me to a life changing journey of self-healing (and tolerance to scent!).

When Michele introduced me to her Energy Release Points as a tool for working through soul issues, it was immediately clear that they are as essential as the Flower Essences Repertory book by Patricia Kaminsky and Richard Katz. My children and I have experienced relief from from a myriad of physical and emotional complaints when we have activated them to resolve soul issues. The Energy Release Points are an invaluable tool; incorporating them into my Colourtouch and Lightbody work has tremendously increased my ability to self heal as I continue my journey toward Ascension."

Pamela Loong - RN BScN - Edmonton AB

"When we carry physical pain in the body, it has been my understanding that sometimes it's associated with an energetic block held trapped in the body. When working with Michele on my own energetic blocks, she introduced me to a method that looks at accessing the Energy Release Points. After my first session and treatment with her tapping into these various access points in the Meridian system, I could feel the energetic block dissipating. I've gone to chiropractic, physiotherapist, and massage therapy, and although they help maintain pain control, nothing has completely worked as well or as fast as tapping into the Energy Release Points, as Michele has done with her treatments. The use of toning into the Energy Release Points with the various frequencies gives it an extra boost to push the energy block out of the body. There are a number of other methods she uses along with doing the inner work on ones self that compliments the Energy Release Point therapy (i.e. Soundtouch, Colourtouch, personal soul searching, past life therapy, purging out the issues that no longer serve our highest good, looking at belief systems, using flower, crystal and star essences to bring forth a more balanced individual). I highly recommend this form of work and am happy she is releasing a book to share how this can be done for others to learn how to move through their own energetic work. I am forever grateful for being connected with her and will continue to work with and support her work, she is a great teacher!"

Mitakuye Oyasin - Jody Donald Senior Manager of
Life Skills, BSW, Visual Artist. Enoch, Alberta

Bibliography and Suggested Reading

Andrews, Ted. <u>Animal-Speak The Spiritual & Magical Powers of Creatures Great & Small.</u> St. Paul, MN USA: Llewellyn Publications, 1999.

Beinfield, Harriet & Korngold, Efrem. <u>Between Heaven and Earth a Guide to Chinese Medicine.</u> New York, NY: The Random House Publishing Group, 1991

Campbell, Joseph. <u>Creative Mythology The Masks of God.</u> New York, NY USA: Penguin Group, 1968.

Case, Paul Foster. <u>The Tarot</u>. Los Angeles, CA USA: Builders of the Adytum, 1990.

Copenhaver, Brian P. <u>Hermetica.</u> Cambridge, UK: Cambridge University Press, 1992.

Cousto, Hans. <u>The Cosmic Octave</u>. Mendocino, CA USA: Life Rhythm Publication, 1988.

Deadman, Peter, & Mazin Al Khafaji w/Kevin Baker. <u>A Manual of Acupuncture</u>. East Sussex, England: Journal of Chinese Medicine Publications, 1998.

Ellis, Andrew, Nigel Wiseman, Ken Boss. <u>Grasping the Wind</u>. Brookline, MA USA: Paradigm Publications, 1989.

Erdoes, Richard & Ortiz, Alfonso. <u>American Indian Myths and Legends.</u> New York, NY USA: Pantheon Books, 1984.

Feng, Gia-Fu, English, Jane. <u>Tao Te Ching.</u> New York, NY USA: Random House 1972

Hurtak, J.J. <u>The Book of Knowledge: The Keys of Enoch.</u> Los Gatos, CA USA: The Academy For Future Science, 1977.

Jarrett, Lonny S. <u>Nourishing Destiny The Inner Tradition of Chinese Medicine.</u> Stockbridge, MA USA: Spirit Path Press, 2000.

Jarrett, Lonny S. <u>The Clinical Practice of Chinese Medicine.</u> Stockbridge, MA USA: Spirit Path Press, 2006.

Kaatz, Debra. <u>Characters of Wisdom Taoist Tales of the Acupuncture Points.</u> Soudorgues, France: The Petite Bergerie Press, 2005.

Kaptchuk, O.M.D., Ted. <u>The Web That Has no Weaver: Understanding Chinese Medicine.</u> New York, NY USA: Congdon & Weed, 1983.

Keats, Brian. <u>Betwixt Heaven & Earth.</u> Bowral, Australia: Brian Keats, 1999.

Knott, Inge Rosa. <u>The Theory of Colourtouch.</u> Canada: Inge Rosa Knott, 2013.

Lundy Miranda, Sutton David, Ashton Anthony, Martineau Jason. <u>Quadrivium The Four Classical Liberal Arts of Number, Geometry, Music and Cosmology.</u> New York, NY USA: Wooden Books Ltd/ Bloomsbury, 2010.

Maciocia, Giovanni. The Channels of Acupuncture - Clinical Use of the Secondary Channels and Eight Extraordinary Vessels. London, England: Churchill Livingstone, 2006.

Mulford, Prentice. Thoughts are Things & God in You. Radford, VA: Wilder Publications, 2008.

Prescott, Andrew. Cloud Gate Acupuncture Point Names A Comprehensive Compendium. Lulu

Reichstein, Gail. Wood Becomes Water Chinese Medicine in Everyday Life. New York, NY USA: Kodansha America, Inc., 1998.

Sankey, Mikio. Esoteric Acupuncture Gateway to Expanded Healing Volume 1. Inglewood, CA USA: Mountain Castle Publishing, 1999.

Strehlow, Wighard. Hildegard of Bingen's Spiritual Remedies. Rochester, Vermont USA: Healing Arts Press, 2002.

Three Initiates. The Kybalion. New York, NY USA: Jeremy P. Tarcher/Penguin, 1908, 2008.

Tresidder, Jack. The Complete Dictionary of Symbols in Myth, Art and Literature. London, UK: Duncan Baird Publishers, 2004.

Wu, Zhongxian. Xin Yi Wu Dao Heart-Mind - The Dao of Martial Arts. London, UK: Singing Dragon, 2014.

Index Of Point And Page Number

ST-19	123	SP-7	148	SI-9	175
ST-20	124	SP-8	149	SI-10	175
ST-21	124	SP-9	150	SI-11	176
ST-22	125	SP-10	150	SI-12	177
ST-23	126	SP-11	151	SI-13	178
ST-24	126	SP-12	152	SI-14	178
ST-25	127	SP-13	153	SI-15	179
ST-26	128	SP-14	153	SI-16	179
ST-27	129	SP-15	154	SI-17	180
ST-28	129	SP-16	155	SI-18	180
ST-29	130	SP-17	156	SI-19	181
ST-30	131	SP-18	157		
ST-31	131	SP-19	158	UB-1	184
ST-32	132	SP-20	158	UB-2	184
ST-33	133	SP-21	159	UB-3	185
ST-34	133			UB-4	186
ST-35	134	HT-1	162	UB-5	187
ST-36	135	HT-2	162	UB-6	187
ST-37	136	HT-3	163	UB-7	188
ST-38	137	HT-4	163	UB-8	189
ST-39	137	HT-5	164	UB-9	189
ST-40	138	HT-6	165	UB-10	190
ST-41	138	HT-7	165	UB-11	191
ST-42	139	HT-8	166	UB-12	191
ST-43	140	HT-9	166	UB-13	192
ST-44	141			UB-14	192
ST-45	141	SI-1	170	UB-15	193
		SI-2	170	UB-16	193
SP-1	144	SI-3	171	UB-17	194
SP-2	145	SI-4	172	UB-18	195
SP-3	145	SI-5	172	UB-19	195
SP-4	146	SI-6	173	UB-20	196
SP-5	147	SI-7	174	UB-21	196
SP-6	148	SI-8	174	UB-22	197

UB-23	197	*UB-57*	219	*KID-23*	245
UB-24	198	*UB-58*	220	*KID-24*	246
UB-25	198	*UB-59*	221	*KID-25*	246
UB-26	199	*UB-60*	221	*KID-26*	247
UB-27	200	*UB-61*	222	*KID-27*	248
UB-28	200	*UB-62*	223		
UB-29	201	*UB-63*	224	*P-1*	250
UB-30	202	*UB-64*	225	*P-2*	250
UB-31	203	*UB-65*	225	*P-3*	251
UB-32	203	*UB-66*	226	*P-4*	251
UB-33	204	*UB-67*	227	*P-5*	252
UB-34	205			*P-6*	252
UB-35	205	*KID-1*	230	*P-7*	253
UB-36	206	*KID-2*	230	*P-8*	254
UB-37	206	*KID-3*	231	*P-9*	254
UB-38	207	*KID-4*	232		
UB-39	208	*KID-5*	233	*TH-1*	258
UB-40	208	*KID-6*	233	*TH-2*	258
UB-41	209	*KID-7*	234	*TH-3*	259
UB-42	209	*KID-8*	235	*TH-4*	260
UB-43	210	*KID-9*	235	*TH-5*	260
UB-44	211	*KID-10*	236	*TH-6*	261
UB-45	211	*KID-11*	237	*TH-7*	261
UB-46	212	*KID-12*	237	*TH-8*	262
UB-47	213	*KID-13*	238	*TH-9*	263
UB-48	213	*KID-14*	239	*TH-10*	263
UB-49	214	*KID-15*	239	*TH-11*	264
UB-50	215	*KID-16*	240	*TH-12*	265
UB-51	216	*KID-17*	241	*TH-13*	265
UB-52	216	*KID-18*	242	*TH-14*	266
UB-53	217	*KID-19*	242	*TH-15*	266
UB-54	218	*KID-20*	243	*TH-16*	267
UB-55	218	*KID-21*	244	*TH-17*	267
UB-56	219	*KID-22*	244	*TH-18*	268

TH-19	268	GB-29	292	DFM-3	324
TH-20	269	GB-30	292	DFM-4	325
TH-21	269	GB-31	293	DFM-5	326
TH-22	270	GB-32	294	DFM-6	326
TH-23	270	GB-33	294	DFM-7	327
		GB-34	295	DFM-8	327
GB-1	274	GB-35	295	DFM-9	328
GB-2	274	GB-36	296	DFM-10	328
GB-3	275	GB-37	297	DFM-11	329
GB-4	276	GB-38	297	DFM-12	329
GB-5	276	GB-39	298	DFM-13	330
GB-6	277	GB-40	299	DFM-14	330
GB-7	277	GB-41	300	DFM-15	331
GB-8	278	GB-42	301	DFM-16	331
GB-9	278	GB-43	302	DFM-17	332
GB-10	279	GB-44	303	DFM-18	333
GB-11	280			DFM-19	333
GB-12	280	LIV-1	306	DFM-20	334
GB-13	281	LIV-2	306	DFM-21	334
GB-14	282	LIV-3	307	DFM-22	335
GB-15	282	LIV-4	308	DFM-23	336
GB-16	283	LIV-5	308	DFM-24	336
GB-17	284	LIV-6	309		
GB-18	284	LIV-7	310	DMD-1	339
GB-19	285	LIV-8	311	DMD-2	340
GB-20	285	LIV-9	311	DMD-3	340
GB-21	286	LIV-10	312	DMD-4	341
GB-22	287	LIV-11	312	DMD-5	342
GB-23	287	LIV-12	313	DMD-6	342
GB-24	288	LIV-13	313	DMD-7	343
GB-25	289	LIV-14	314	DMD-8	343
GB-26	290			DMD-9	344
GB-27	290	DFM-1	323	DMD-10	344
GB-28	291	DFM-2	324	DMD-11	345